ESSENTIAL USES

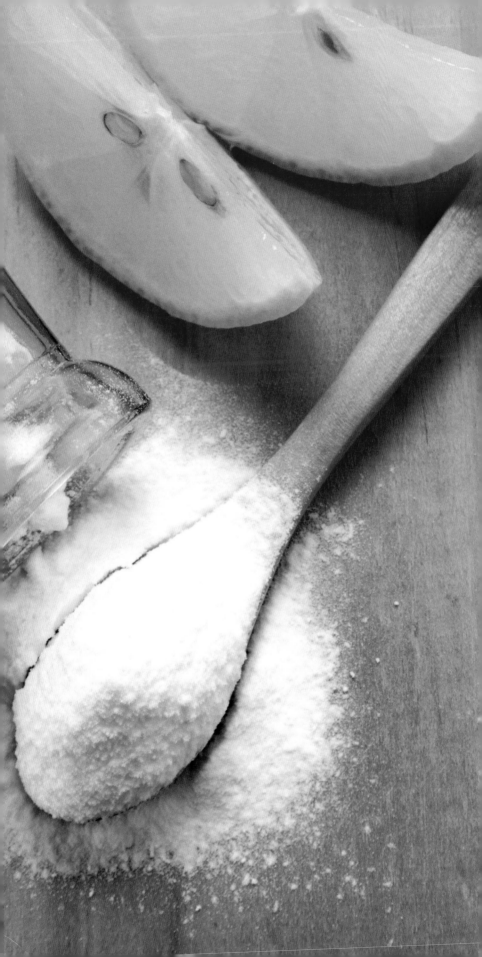

ESSENTIAL USES

BAKING SODA, SALT, VINEGAR, LEMON, COCONUT OIL, HONEY, and GINGER

The ultimate wellness,
beauty, and healthy-home bible

Tricia Swanton

ThunderBay
P·R·E·S·S

San Diego, California

Thunder Bay Press
An imprint of Printers Row Publishing Group
10350 Barnes Canyon Road, Suite 100, San Diego, CA 92121
www.thunderbaybooks.com

Copyright © 2019 Thunder Bay Press

Thunder Bay Press
Publisher: Peter Norton
Associate Publisher: Ana Parker
Publishing/Editorial Team: April Farr, Vicki Jaeger, Kelly Larsen, Stephanie Romero, Kathryn C. Dalby, Carrie Davis
Editorial Team: JoAnn Padgett, Melinda Allman
Production Team: Jonathan Lopes, Rusty von Dyl

Produced by Moseley Road Inc., www.moseleyroad.com
President: Sean Moore
Production Director: Adam Moore
Cover Designer: Lisa Purcell
Supplemental Writers: Grace Moore, Finn Moore, Nancy J. Hajeski

Library of Congress Cataloging-in-Publication data is available upon request.

ISBN: 978-1-68412-638-5

Printed in China

23 22 21 20 19   1 2 3 4 5

CONTENTS

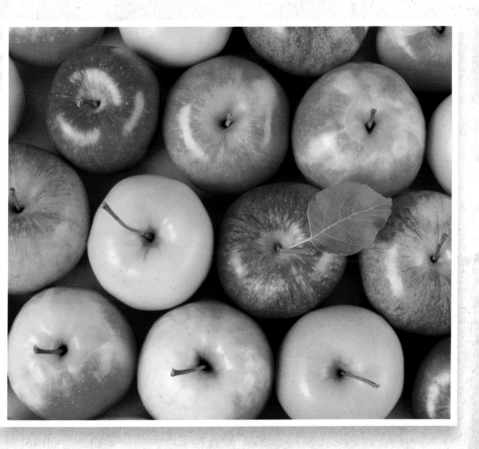

USING NATURAL INGREDIENTS

There are a thousand man-made products you can buy to deal with just about any problem you might come across, from cleaning your house to exfoliating your skin. Some of those products might even work! But, when it comes down to it, the costs almost always outweigh the benefits. When you buy a synthetic household cleaner or body wash, you might get the job done, but you'll also be spending far too much money and using a product that introduces harsh, environmentally harmful chemicals into your home and your body.

GET MORE FOR LESS

There is, of course, another option. Instead of wasting your money, damaging the environment, and putting your own health at risk, you can get the same—or better—results out of things that you probably already have around the house for a fraction of the cost. With nothing but the liberal application of common household items like lemon juice, apple cider vinegar, and coconut oil, you can make great improvements to all aspects of your life.

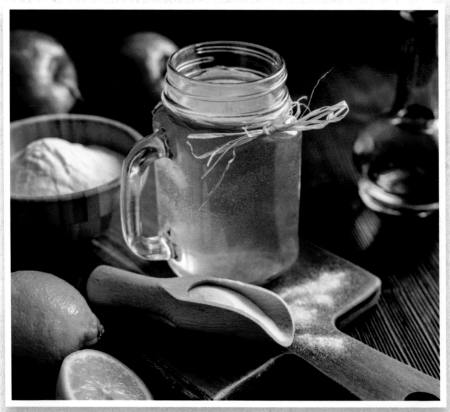

Detox drink made of water, apple cider vinegar, lemon juice, and baking soda (above); coconut oil and coconuts (opposite)

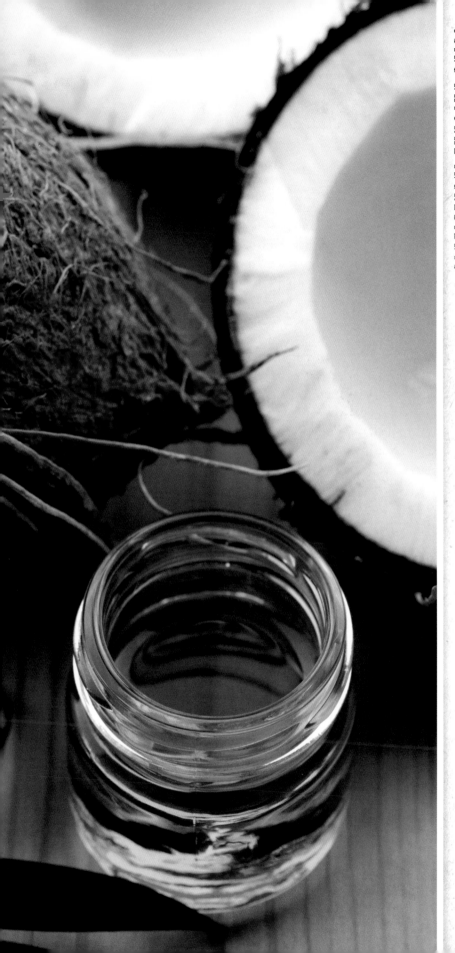

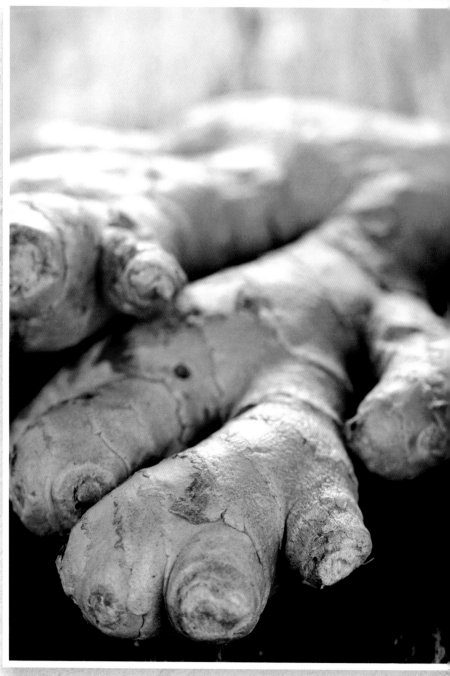

Fresh and ground ginger root

In this book, you will learn new ways to use baking soda, salt, vinegar, lemons, coconut oil, honey, ginger, and a myriad of other natural items. Baking soda makes a perfect alternative to most man-made cleaning solutions, and is gentle enough to avoid damaging surfaces. Salt is rich in vitamins and minerals that are vital for your body's health, and also makes a great exfoliant to help soften and rejuvenate your skin. Apple cider vinegar can help cure dandruff, improve your digestive health, and even remove warts. Lemon juice can be used to freshen your breath and whiten your teeth, while both coconut oil and honey are great for you skin, hair, and overall health. Ginger is as close as you

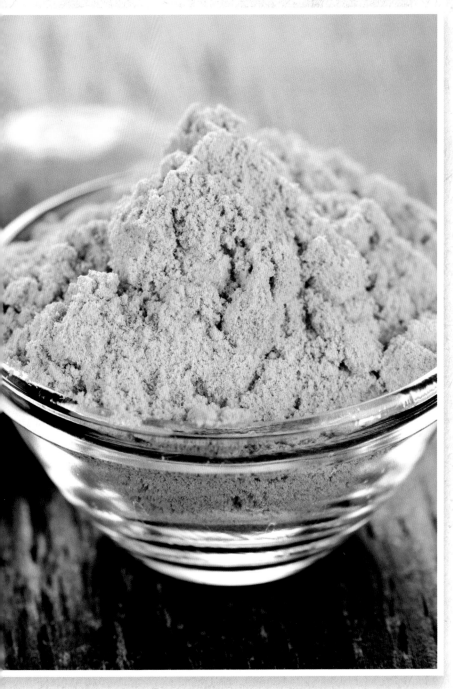

can get to a superfood; you can add it to your diet to help fight off disease, or add it to a face or body mask to cleanse and soften your skin.

MAKE IT YOURSELF
Also included in this book are countless recipes, instructions, and tips to help you create your own DIY face masks, bath salts, and soothing herbal teas, all using nothing but these natural ingredients that you can find around the home or in any store near you. By making use of the information in this book, you can start to take better care of your skin, your health, and your home—all

while saving money, getting better results out of your products, and reducing the overall harm you do to the environment.

Every one of these natural items has its own benefits, and once you learn the best ways to put them to use, you will be able to start cutting out toxic and expensive chemical products from your life, replacing them instead with green, natural solutions that provide all the same benefits with none of the harmful side effects or carbon footprint. From using dark chocolate to help kick your caffeine addiction to using ground cloves to prevent wrinkles and liver spots, there's something here for anyone who wants to start taking steps towards living a healthier, more natural life.

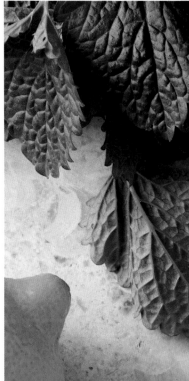

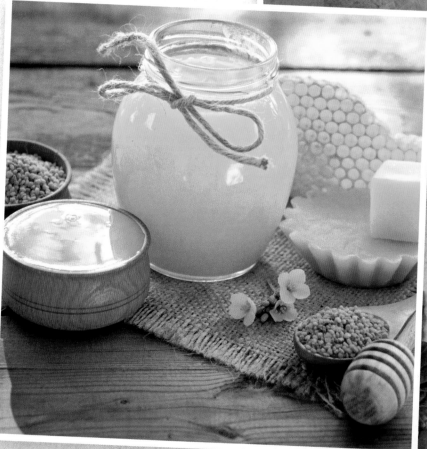

Honey, honeycomb, honey candles, and bee pollen (above); lemon balm tea with honey (opposite)

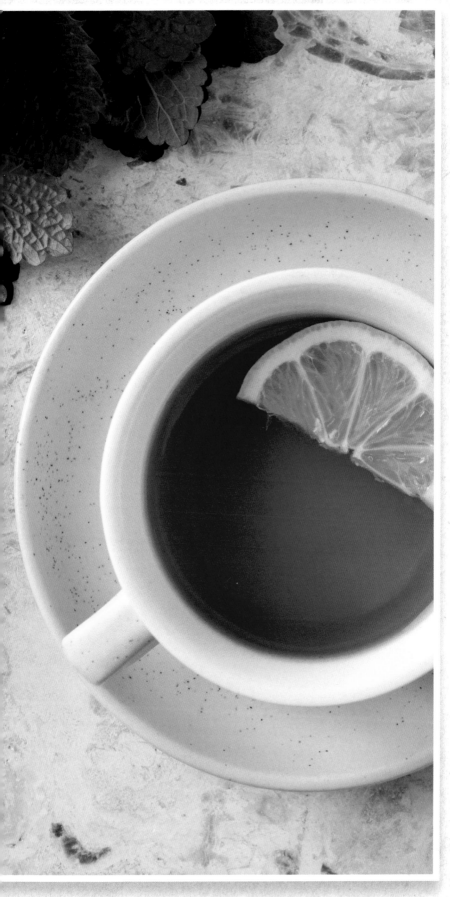

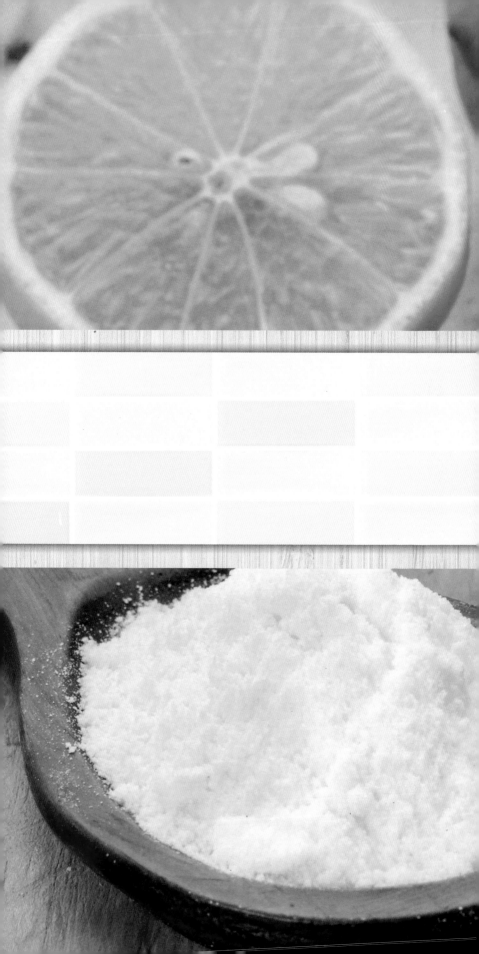

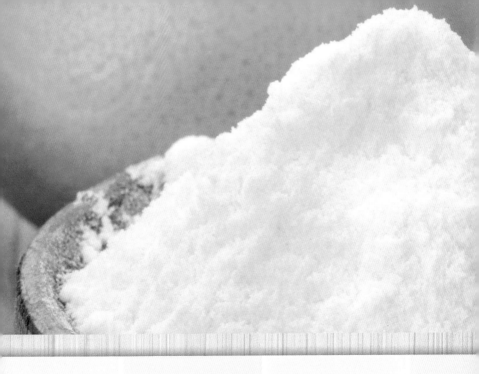

CHAPTER 1
BAKING SODA

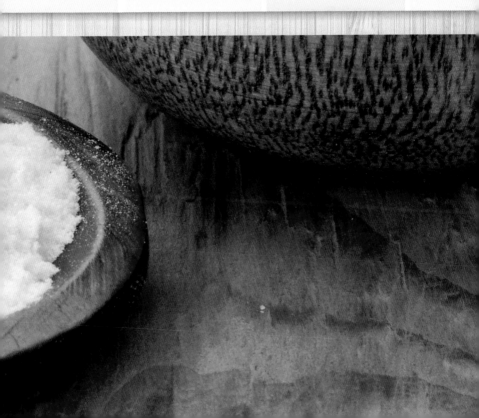

BAKING SODA USES

Baking soda, or sodium bicarbonate, is a mineral found and mined around the world. Throughout history, baking soda has been used as a leavening agent in baking, as it causes batter to rise. Baking soda has a variety of uses that can benefit your health, home, and general wellness. A popular addition to most kitchen cupboards, it has invaluable uses in cooking and cleaning, as well as being an inexpensive remedy for many common ailments.

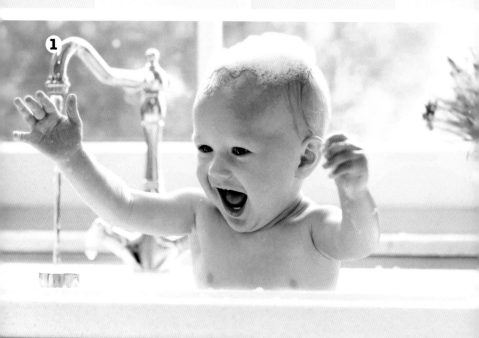

1 Baking soda
   in your baby's
   bathwater
2 Soothe poison
   ivy rash
3 Paste of baking
   soda and water
   for bug bites
4 Hand scrub with
   baking soda and
   honey
5 Baking soda
   toothpaste
6 Polish tarnished
   jewelry

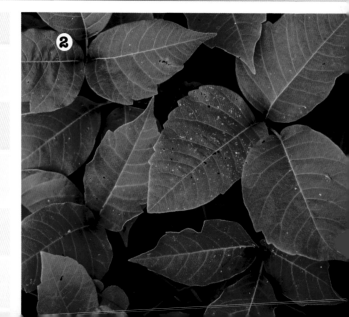

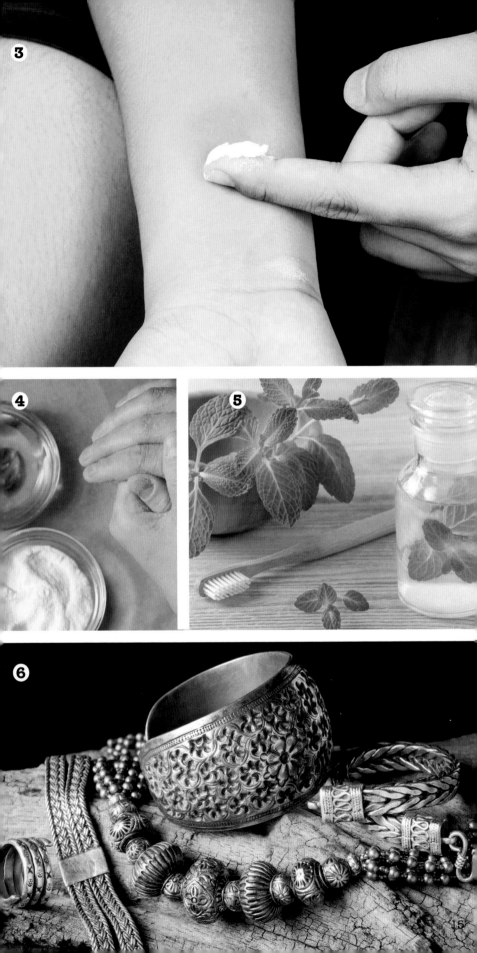

WELLNESS

Aside from its uses in baking, baking soda is best known for its natural cleaning abilities. While it is an incredibly effective, inexpensive, and versatile cleaning agent, it also boasts a wide variety of wellness benefits.

From calming irritated skin to upset stomachs, baking soda can go a long way in keeping your family healthy. Baking soda is very alkaline, meaning its makeup has the properties of an alkali and is very basic. It is this alkalinity that makes it such an effective levener in baking Because of its basic pH level, baking soda can neutralize stomach acids quickly to counter any digestive issues. Additionally, baking soda is lightly abrasive and is therefore a gentle way to clean your teeth and body.

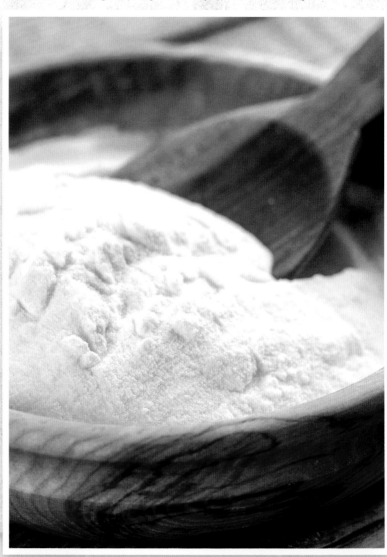

CALM INSECT BITES AND STINGS

Make a paste of baking soda and water and apply to your skin. Apply the paste up to three times a day. This is an effective method to combat itchy bites as well as painful bee and wasp stings.

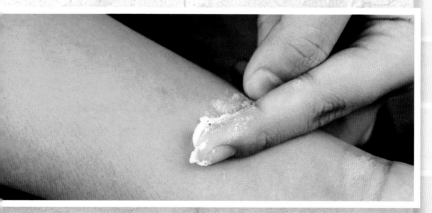

Baking soda and water paste for itchy bites

NATURAL MOUTHWASH

Rinsing your mouth with baking soda mouthwash daily helps to treat and prevent halitosis, discourage the formation of plaque, prevent gum disease, and maintain a healthy oral pH balance. If you have a canker sore, rinsing your mouth every few hours with this solution will help to heal the sore faster and alleviate some of the pain.

To make the mouthwash, mix 1 teaspoon baking soda into a glass of water and stir until the baking soda is dissolved.

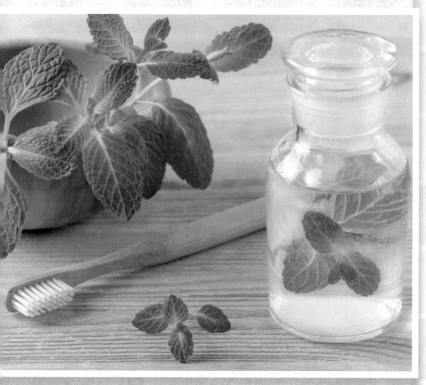

Baking soda and mint to make mouthwash

WELLNESS

RELIEVE HEARTBURN

Baking soda is a safe antacid—it can help to neutralize acid buildup and improve pH balance in the body. To help heartburn from eating acidic foods, slowly drink ¼ teaspoon baking soda dissolved in a glass of water to neutralize the acid and correct your body's pH balance.

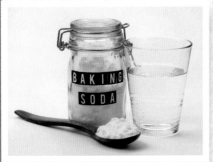

SOOTHE IRRITATED SKIN

Add 1 cup baking soda to bathwater to soften your skin and relieve irritation. Two tablespoons baking soda added to your baby's bathwater can relieve diaper rash.

To counter more aggressive irritations, make a paste of equal parts baking soda and water and apply it to skin affected by poison ivy and poison oak to reduce discomfort. Do not use this method on broken skin. The paste also works for skin affected by sunburn and rashes caused by allergic reactions. Leave this mixture on the skin for several minutes before rinsing. Repeat a few times per day as needed.

WARNING!
When it comes to ingesting baking soda, less is more! Consuming too much baking soda can cause an increase in acid production.

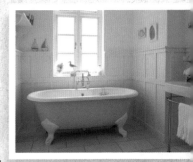

Add baking soda to bath water

REMOVE SPLINTERS

If you have a stubborn splinter, try soaking the area in baking soda and water. Mix 1 tablespoon baking soda with warm water and soak the area twice a day. Using this method, splinters will come out naturally after a few sessions.

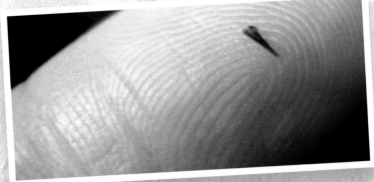

BOOST YOUR WORKOUTS

You can use baking soda before and after your workouts in order to get the most out of them. Some studies indicate that baking soda reduces post-workout fatigue and potentially enhances athletic performance when taken before a workout. The ideal dosage of baking soda as a pre-working supplement is 135 mg of baking soda per pound of body weight.

Mix the baking soda with warm water and stir until the baking soda is completely dissolved. Drink the mixture slowly, about 90–120 minutes before your workout for best results.

Tip: Combine with 0.3 ounces creatine per pound of body weight in order to enhance its benefits. Creatine is a nitrogenous organic acid that is found naturally in muscle cells and is a popular supplement amongst athletes.

WARNING!

Baking soda is SODIUM bicarbonate; be aware of its effects if you are avoiding sodium for health reasons

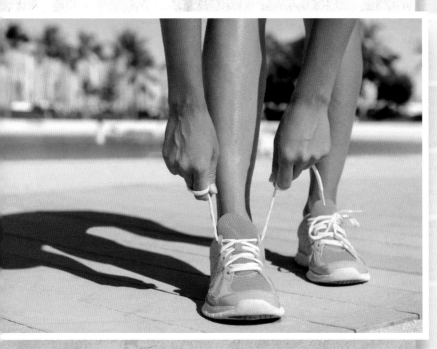

IMPROVE KIDNEY FUNCTION

Baking soda buffers acids in the body and helps to keep pH levels balanced. Consuming baking soda can help with removing acid from the body and research has suggested it may slow the progress of chronic kidney disease in some cases.

Be sure to speak to your doctor if you are interested in any baking soda treatment for kidney disease.

WARNING!
Always consult a doctor before drinking baking soda and water.

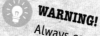

BEAUTY/PERSONAL

Baking soda is an antifungal and an antiseptic, making it a wonderful natural answer to many beauty questions.

Baking soda is mildly abrasive and will gently exfoliate your face, feet, hands, and body. Additionally, baking soda's ability to absorb and prevent odors makes it a natural alternative to deodorant on its own, as well as being the perfect main ingredient for DIY deodorants. Its antifungal and abrasive qualities also make it an important element of maintaining good oral hygiene. Whether you're in pursuit of white teeth, healthier hair, or smoother skin, baking soda is the inexpensive and natural ingredient that can help you achieve your beauty goals.

GENTLY EXFOLIATE FACE AND BODY
Mix 3 parts baking soda with 1 part water, rub gently in a circular motion, and rinse clean.

SOOTHE SORE FEET
Create a footbath with 1 tablespoon baking soda and warm water. Soaking your feet in this mixture will remove bacteria and odors, can help prevent toenail fungus, and can also soften calluses that cause pain or discomfort.

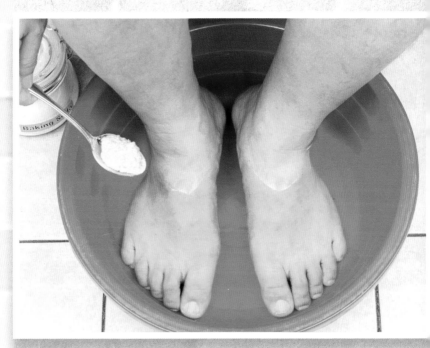

Soak your feet in baking soda

CLEAN YOUR MAKEUP BRUSHES

Soak your brushes in a solution of 1 teaspoon baking soda and 1 cup water. This will remove any oils, buildup, and residue on your brushes. **Tip:** This process will also work for your hairbrush and combs!

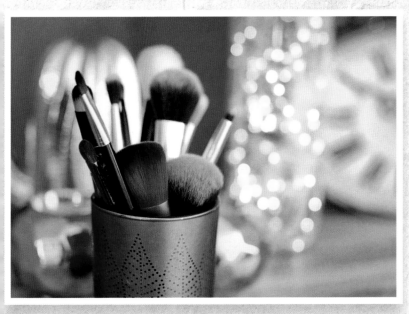

BRUSH YOUR TEETH

Many commercial toothpastes contain potentially harmful ingredients such as triclosan and sodium lauryl sulfate, as well as others that are more controversial, such as fluoride, propylene glycol, and sodium hydroxide. If you would like more control over what goes into your body, making your own toothpaste is incredibly easy and is beneficial both for yourself and the environment.

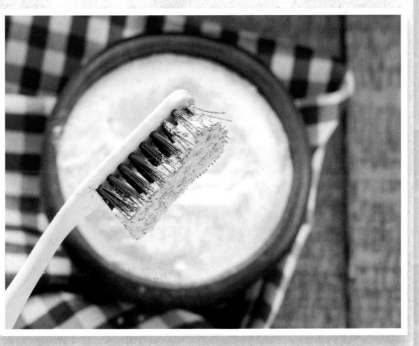

BEAUTY/PERSONAL

Using natural ingredients in your toothpaste is an easy way to guarantee good oral hygiene while controlling what's going into your body. Here are two recipes for natural toothpaste you can make at home.

Coconut Oil Toothpaste

2 tablespoons coconut oil
1 tablespoon baking soda
1 tablespoon sea salt, finely ground
1–2 drops essential oil, or to taste (optional)

Place coconut oil into a glass bowl. Set that bowl in hot water to liquify the coconut oil. While the oil is melting, measure dry ingredients into a separate bowl and mix. Add coconut oil and essential oils to your dry ingredients and mix thoroughly until blended. Store the finished product in a lidded glass jar at room temperature.

WARNING!
There is some concern that baking soda can be too abrasive for everyday use, so find the balance of baking soda and salt that's right for you!

Hydrogen Peroxide Toothpaste

2 tablespoons baking soda
1 tablespoon 3% hydrogen peroxide
½ tablespoon sea salt, finely ground (optional)
1–2 drops essential oil, or to taste (optional)

Combine dry ingredients in a small bowl and mix. Add essential oil and hydrogen peroxide. Stir until a smooth, thick paste forms. Store your finished product in a lidded glass jar at room temperature.
Tip: Try adding ½ teaspoon activated charcoal powder for an extra whitening boost.

The antibacterial properties of coconut oil help reduce plaque and stains, while baking soda alkalizes acid in the mouth and helps to remove plaque and stains, and activated charcoal's natural adhesive qualities let it bind with surface-staining culprits and take them off your teeth. Add a drop or two of essential oils for that minty-fresh taste to create a cheap, easy-to-use toothpaste that's made up of natural ingredients.

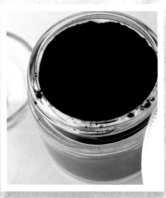

Charcoal powder

MAKE DEODORANT

Many deodorants and antiperspirants contain ingredients that are detrimental to your health, including aluminum, parabens, propylene glycol, phthalates, and triclosan. Aluminum in particular has been the subject of several studies on antiperspirants; it is suggested that the chemicals in your antiperspirant are absorbed into the skin and a few studies have theorized that aluminum-based antiperspirants may increase the risk for breast cancer.

Luckily, there is a healthy, cost-effective alternative that you can make yourself! Make your own deodorant using baking soda to keep yourself smelling fresh without harming your body.

FYI: Going Camping?

Ditch your old toothpaste. The mint flavoring in commercial toothpaste can attract bears! Bring your newly-made toothpaste to keep your teeth clean and keep you safe (but hold off on the essential oils).

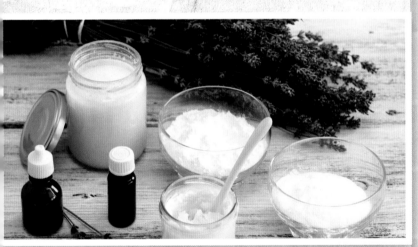

Mix your ingredients to make deodorant

Natural Deodorant

1 cup coconut oil
2 tablespoons baking soda
1 cup arrowroot powder or organic cornstarch
10–15 drops essential oils, or to preference

Combine all ingredients in a small bowl and mix until blended. If you have sensitive skin, apply your new deodorant on a small patch of skin to test for any allergic reactions. Apply deodorant to your underarms with your fingers and wait for it to dry to avoid getting any on your clothes.
Tip: You can purchase empty deodorant sticks to fill with your natural deodorant, but be sure to store it in the fridge during the warmer months to avoid the coconut oil melting.

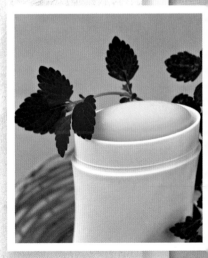

BEAUTY/PERSONAL

WASH YOUR HAIR

Your hair contains natural oil, which gives your hair its shine and keeps it healthy and conditioned. Many commercial shampoos contain chemical additives such as sodium lauryl sulfate, sodium laureth sulfate, fragrance, and cocamide DEA, all of which have been linked to hair damage as well as other more serious side effects. These will strip healthy oils from your hair, leaving it dry and brittle. Additionally, overwashing your hair combined with the use of shampoo can actually worsen dandruff and cause an overproduction of oil, making your hair greasy much faster.

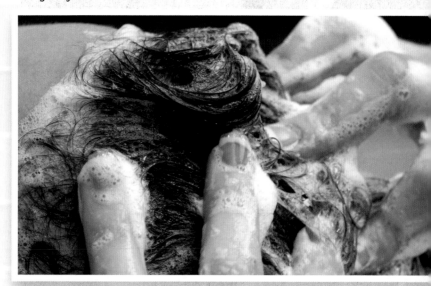

Scrub your scalp

Baking Soda and Vinegar Shampoo

1 cup baking soda, 3 cups water
2 cups apple cider vinegar, 4 cups water

Mix the baking soda and water together and store in a squeeze bottle. Mix the apple cider vinegar and water mixture and store in a separate squeeze bottle. Apply baking soda mixture to dry or wet hair, starting at the roots and working towards the ends. Let sit for 1–3 minutes then rinse with water. Rinse hair with vinegar mixture, then rinse with water.

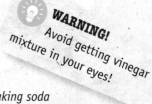

WARNING!
Avoid getting vinegar mixture in your eyes!

Tip: If the vinegar mixture is too harsh for your hair type, try adding an extra cup of water to dilute the mixture further.

NOTE:
Baking soda can damage your hair if used too regularly. It is recommended that you use this shampoo mixture once a week, with more regular vinegar rinses.

BRIGHTEN YOUR JEWELRY

Remove tarnish from your silver jewelry by making a paste of three parts baking soda to one part water. Apply with a lint-free cloth and rinse.

Tip: Avoid using paper towels to apply the mixture, as they can scratch the surfaces of your jewelry.

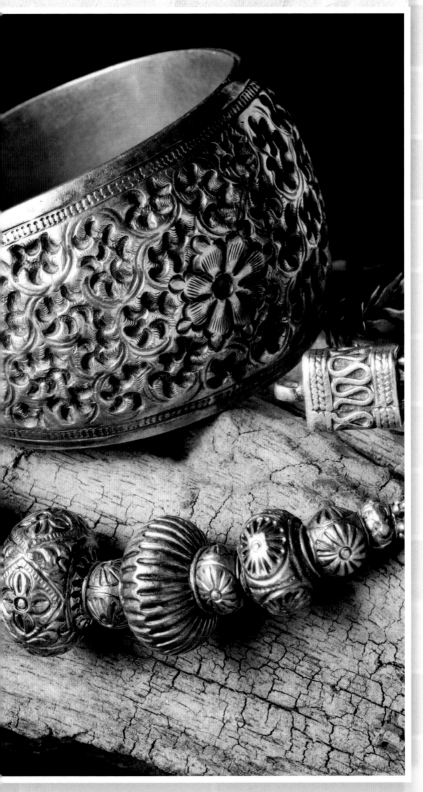

BEAUTY/PERSONAL

MAKE A FACE MASK

If your skin is feeling tired, try making a natural face mask with baking soda, honey, and lemon. Baking soda can be anti-inflammatory and antibacterial, while honey can moisturize your skin and lemon juice can be slightly antibacterial and exfoliating.

Citrus-Honey Mask

WARNING!
Avoid getting vinegar mixture in your eyes!

½ teaspoon lemon juice
½ teaspoon baking soda
1 tablespoon honey

Mix ingredients until smooth. Apply to face and gently spread on the skin, do not rub. Rinse after 15 minutes.

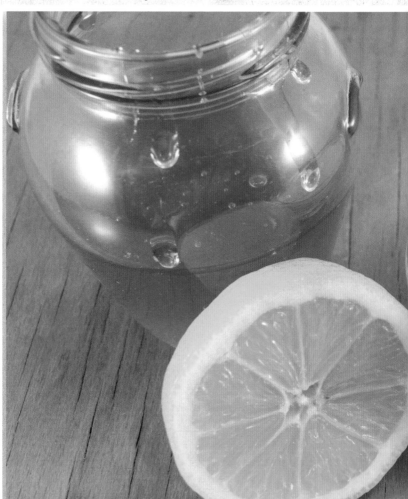

Baking soda with honey and lemon

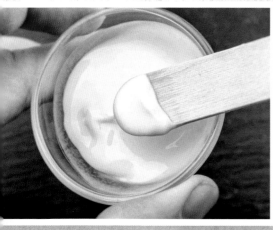

aking soda and water paste

PIMPLE TREATMENT

Mix a small amount of baking soda and water to make a thick paste. Apply to the pimple, let it sit for 15 minutes, and rinse off with warm water.

Tip: Apply with a cotton swab to avoid touching your face and potentially worsening the breakout.

WARNING!
Don't use this method too often, as it can dry the skin.

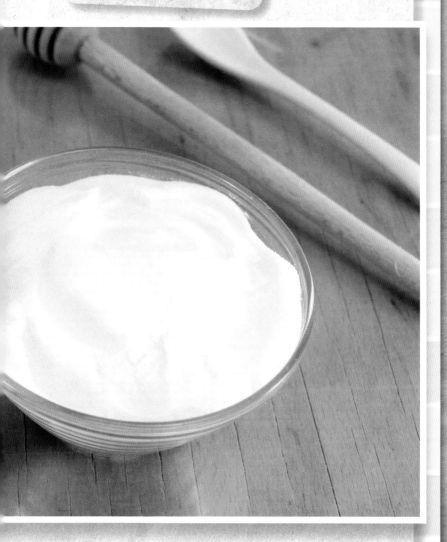

HOME

Many commercial cleaning agents—whether it be window cleaner, kitchen cleaning products, furniture polish, or even fabric softener—can contain chemicals that are harmful for your own health as well as the health of your children and pets.

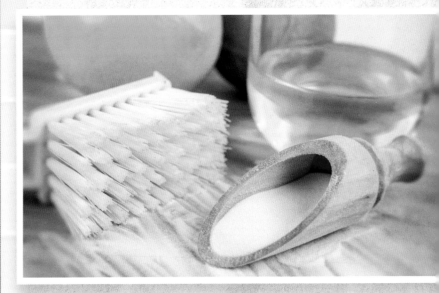

Clean with baking soda

Baking soda is an incredibly effective abrasive while still being gentle enough to not damage any surfaces in your home. It is also a great natural deodorizer that can be utilized anywhere from your mattress to your fridge to your carpets. Whether used alone or in combination with other household basics, baking soda is the natural cleaning solution to your household messes.

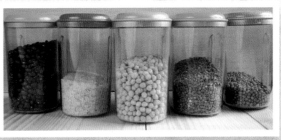

KITCHEN
Remove stains from plastic containers
Wipe your food containers with a clean sponge sprinkled with baking soda. For tougher stains, soak the containers in a solution of four teaspoons baking soda to 1 quart warm water.

Freshen up your fridge

Baking soda will absorb strong food odors—try leaving some baking soda in the back of your fridge.

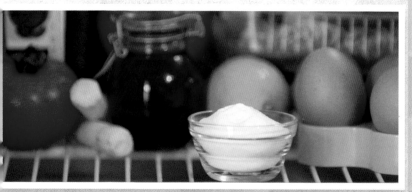

Bowl of baking soda in fridge

Clean your kitchen surfaces

Sprinkle baking soda onto a clean damp sponge or cloth and clean as usual. Rinse thoroughly and wipe dry. This method is safe on all kitchen surfaces.

Tip: For a deeper clean, make a paste with baking soda, coarse salt, and liquid dish soap to scour tough grime.

Tip 2: Polish the surfaces with a cloth dampened with white vinegar and water to remove any streaks left by the baking soda.

Degrease dishes and pans

Add a sprinkle of baking soda to a pan for dissolving stuck-on grease.

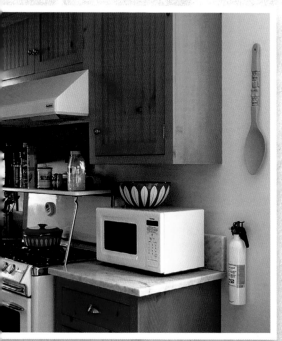

Fire Extinguisher

Pouring baking soda on a small pan fire should stifle the flames quickly. It's always a good idea to keep a fire extinguisher in your kitchen, but baking soda will do for a minor grease fire.

Tip: Never pour water on a grease fire!

Keep a fire extinguisher in your kitchen

HOME

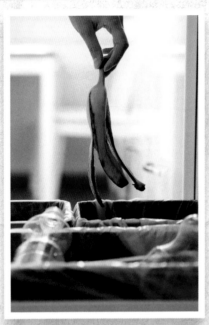

Baking soda to eliminate odors

Deodorize your garbage can
Pour baking soda into the bottom of your trash can to fight odors.

Clean your coffeepot
Mix ¼ cup baking soda with 1 quart warm water. Rub the mixture into the pot to remove stains or bad tastes. In the case of tough stains, let the mixture sit for a few hours. Then rinse.

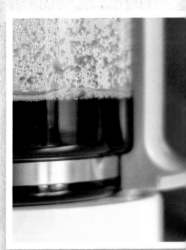

Clean your coffeepot

Clean silverware
Create a paste of three parts baking soda to one part water. Apply this with a lint-free cloth; let sit for 15 to 20 minutes, then rinse.
Tip: Avoid using paper towels to apply the mixture, as they can scratch your silverware.

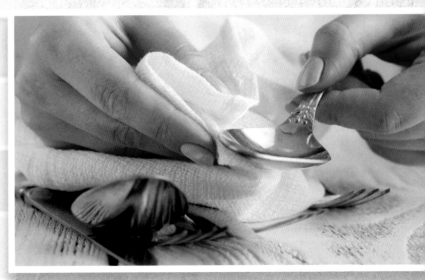

Polish silverware

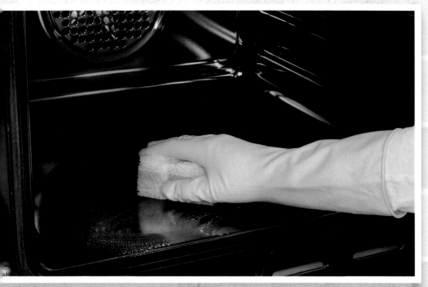

Keep your oven clean

Oven cleaner

Add 1 teaspoon baking soda to a damp rag or sponge to wipe away any food or grease remnants. Rinse well.

Give your dishwasher a hand

By making your own detergent with baking soda, you will eliminate unwanted grease and grime that builds up on your dishes as well as lowering the amount of harmful chemicals used in your home, helping both yourself and the environment.

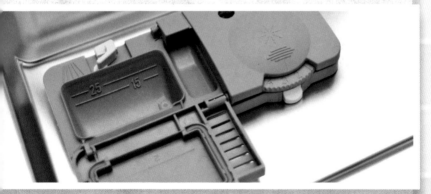

Baking soda in detergent cup

Easy Dishwasher Detergent

3 drops liquid dishwashing soap
Baking soda
Salt

Add 3 drops regular dish soap to your dishwasher's detergent cup, then fill the cup half of the way up with baking soda. Fill the remaining cup space with salt and run your dishwasher as normal.

HOME

DIY: Detergent Pods

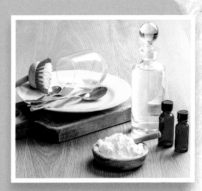

You will need:
1 cup baking soda
1 cup soda ash
1 cup salt
¼ cup citric acid
1 cup water
½ cup white vinegar (per cycle)

Directions:
In a large bowl, mix the baking soda, soda ash, salt, and citric acid. Add the water to the dry ingredients and mix thoroughly. Scoop 1 tablespoon of the mixture into a mold (an ice cube tray works great!) or onto a clean, non-porous surface to create individual detergent pods and let dry overnight. Once dry, store your new detergent pods in an airtight container. Run dishwasher as usual, but be sure to pour ½ cup white vinegar into rinse aid spout before each cycle

Scrub your veggies
Baking soda is a food-safe way to remove any dirt or residue off of fresh fruit and vegetables. Just sprinkle some baking soda onto a damp cloth, wipe your produce, and rinse.

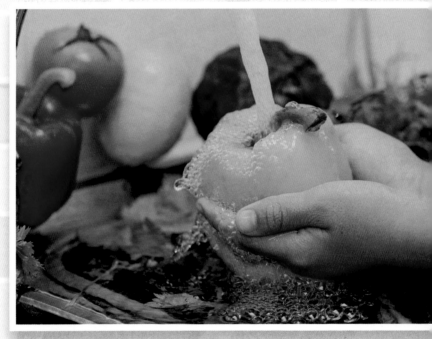

Wash your produce

Fix burned pans

Boil two inches of water in a pan with a burned bottom. Turn off the heat, then add ½ cup baking soda and let soak overnight. The pan should be easy to clean come morning.

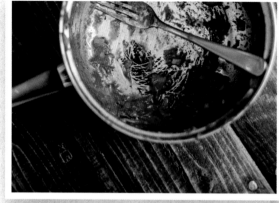

Clean dirty pots

BATH

Remove mildew

Scrub your tub, tile, or sink with a damp sponge and baking soda for a healthy way to keep your bathroom clean.

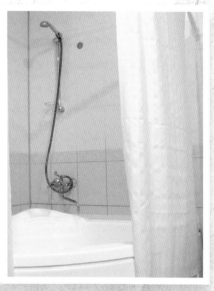

Remove mildew from shower curtains

De-clog a drain

Pour ½ cup baking soda down your drain and follow with ½ cup white vinegar to recreate your school science project in your bathroom. Cover with a wet cloth to contain the reaction. Wait five minutes and then flush with hot water to clear the drain. This method will work on any mild clog.

Shower Curtain Cleaner

Wipe shower curtains with a damp cloth or sponge sprinkled with baking soda and rinse to remove grime and mildew.

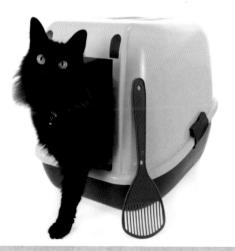

Litter Deodorizer

Cover the bottom of your cat's litter box with baking soda before filling with litter to naturally deodorize your cat box. Sprinkle extra baking soda on top for a deodorizing boost after cleaning out the box.

HOME

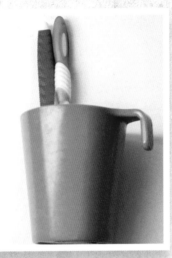

Clean toothbrushes

Clean your toothbrush

Mix 1 teaspoon baking soda with 1 cup warm water. Soak toothbrushes overnight to clean the bristles. Remember to still replace your toothbrush regularly!

Septic care

Flushing 1 cup baking soda per week will keep your septic system functioning well and will maintain a good pH balance in your septic tank.

Clean marble countertops

Sprinkle baking soda onto a clean damp sponge or cloth and clean as usual. Rinse thoroughly and wipe dry. This method is also safe for ceramic bathroom tiles, toilets, showers, bathtubs, and sinks.

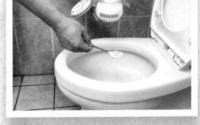

Flush baking soda

Tip: For a deeper clean, make a paste with baking soda. Using a sponge or cloth, rub the mixture onto the surface you want to clean. Let it sit for 15–20 minutes and then wipe with a cloth to scour tough grime.

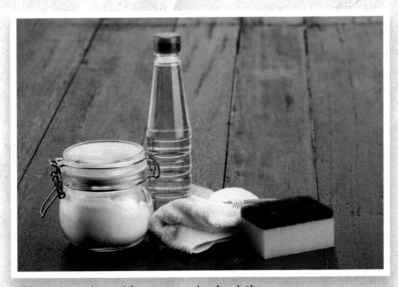

Baking soda can be used for numerous cleaning duties

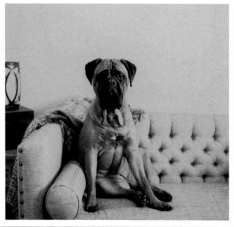

Freshen upholstery

LIVING ROOM
Deodorize musty upholstery
Sprinkle the fabric surfaces of your home with baking soda. Let sit for 15 minutes, then vacuum.

Tip: You can use this method on your mattress as well as your pets' beds.

Remove crayon from walls
Don't want to repaint every time your child decides to move from paper to the walls? Scrub lightly with a damp sponge sprinkled in baking soda to remove crayon marks.

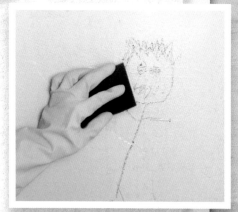

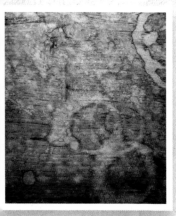

Remove water rings

Buff out water rings
Make a paste of one part baking soda to one part water. Apply this to any water rings left on your wooden surfaces and gently buff the stain away.

Carpet cleaner
Many carpet cleaners contain chemicals that are harmful to children and pets. Baking soda is a natural way to keep your home clean while keeping your family healthy.

Sprinkle your carpet with baking soda; let it sit for 15–20 minutes, then vacuum. For a deeper clean, spray the stained area with a 1:1 mixture of white vinegar and water. Wait up to an hour, or until the surface dries, then scrub the baking soda loose and vacuum.

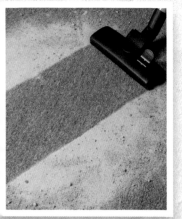

Clean carpets

HOME

All-purpose floor cleaner
This natural floor cleaner is safe for wood and tile floors alike and will remove any lingering smells.

Natural Floor Cleaner

¼ cup white vinegar
¼ cup baking soda
1 teaspoon liquid
dishwashing soap
2 gallons warm water
Tip: Add a few drops of essential oils to increase the mixture's odor-neutralizing power.

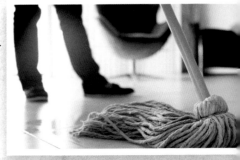
Clean floors

LAUNDRY ROOM

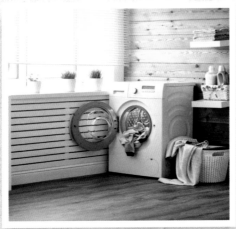
Keep your laundry fresh

Brighten your laundry
Add 1 cup baking soda to your laundry load to brighten whites and colors alike. When combined with liquid detergent, baking soda will help balance pH levels to give clothes a more thorough clean.

Use 1 cup baking soda alone in your laundry for a gentle way to clean and soften baby clothes.

Deodorize sneakers
Sprinkle some baking soda inside your shoes (and your gym bag) to minimize odor. Just be sure to shake out the excess before you put them on next!

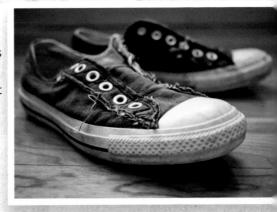
Minimize shoe odor

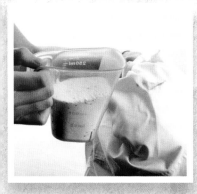

Remove stains

To remove perspiration stains, mix 4 tablespoons baking soda with ¼ cup water into a think paste. Rub the paste into the stain, let it sit for an hour, and launder as usual. This mixture is also effective in removing rust stains and fresh grease stains. For general stain removal, let the baking soda mixture sit for 3 hours before washing.

For fresh coffee and wine stains, soak the area in white vinegar and dab with a clean towel, then sprinkle baking soda over the stain and rub with a clean, soft toothbrush before laundering in cold water.

For oil stains, add a drizzle of dish soap over the baking soda before brushing the stain and laundering in cold water.

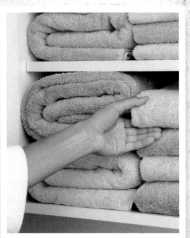

Improve your linen closet

Place an open box or bowl of baking soda in your linen closet to fight musty smells in your sheets and towels.
Tip: This also works for your bedroom closets!

Freshen up your hamper

Sprinkle baking soda into the bottom of your clothes hamper to keep odors away, as a hamper can absorb the odors of what it contains over time.

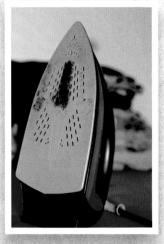

Clean scorch marks from your iron

Clean your iron

In order to not leave stains or marks on your light-colored clothes, give your iron a clean using white vinegar and baking soda.

Soak a piece of paper towel or clean cloth with vinegar, then sprinkle baking soda over the cloth. Place the iron on the cloth and move in circular motions (with the iron off). Once it's clean, turn the iron on the steam setting to remove any baking soda from the iron's holes. Repeat this process until your iron is clean.

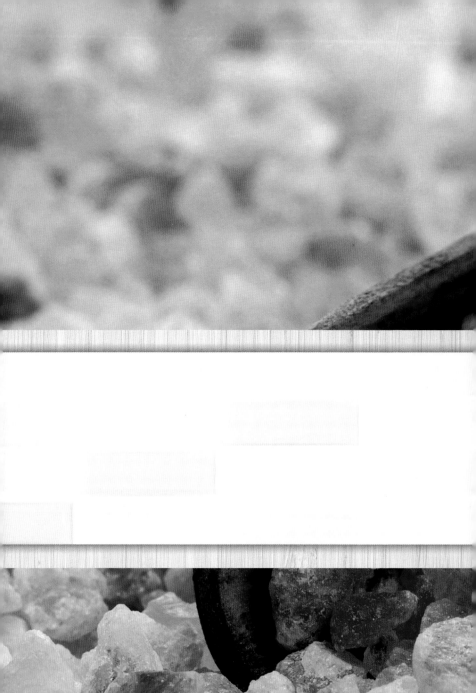

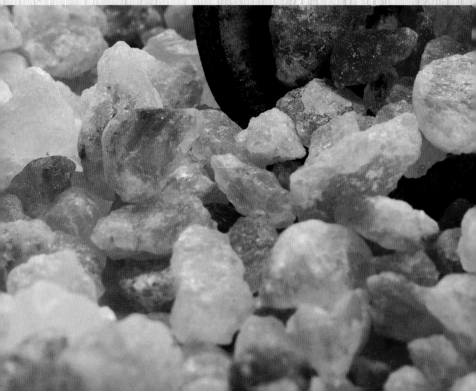

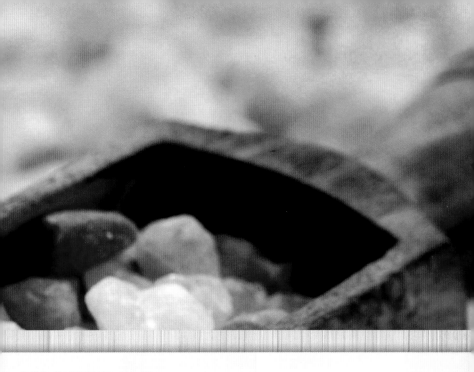

CHAPTER 2
SALT

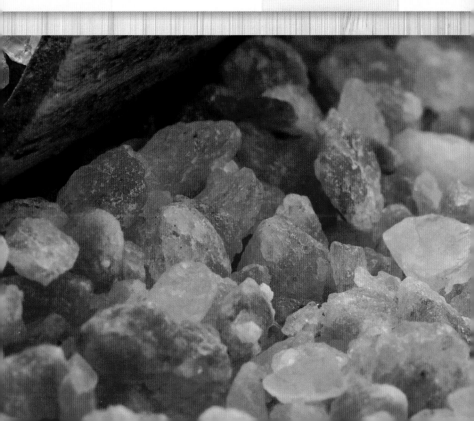

SALT USES

While it is best-known for its presence at the dinner table, salt can be used to great effect in just about every context. This household standard can serve as an affordable and effective component in just about any way you can think of, from cooking meals and cleaning the house to soothing muscle pain and treating insect bites.

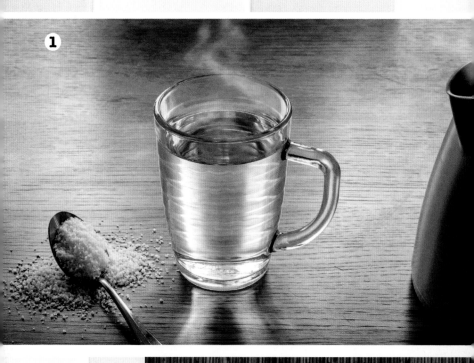

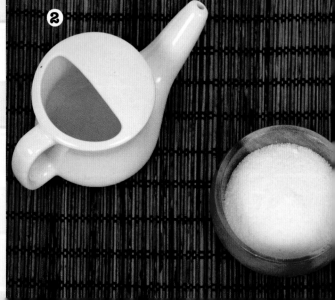

1 Salt water
2 Neti pot with salt
3 Colored bath salts
4 Coarse salt

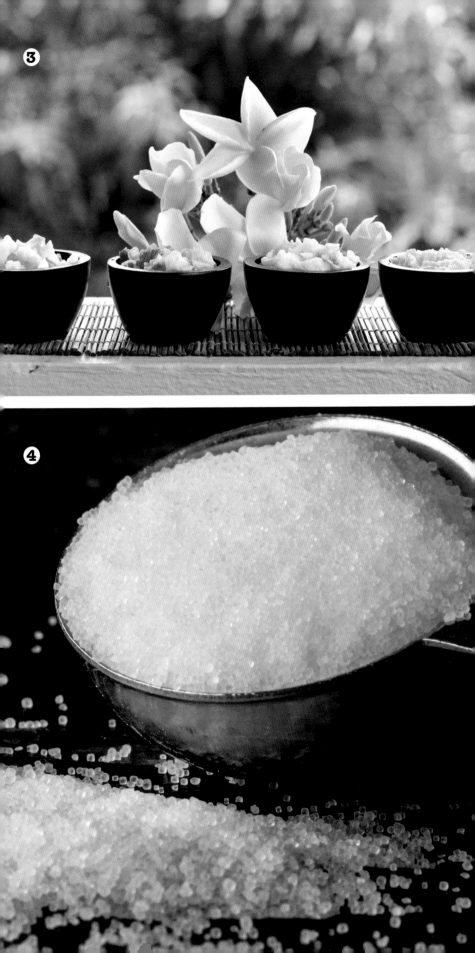

WELLNESS

Maintaining the right amount of salt in your body and diet is a vital aspect of human health. Low salt intake can lead to complications such as poor blood pressure and heart health, iodine deficiency, hypothyroidism, and diabetes. Aside from the health benefits of simply maintaining a healthy amount of salt in your diet, salt has also been used for centuries as a remedy for a countless number of ailments

Because of its antibacterial and anti-inflammatory properties, salt can be used as a home remedy to treat infection, reduce swelling and pain, and improve respiratory health, among many other possible uses.

MEDICINAL SALTS

While standard table salt can serve perfectly well in many cases—and has the added bonus of being edible—other kinds of salts may provide better results when used medicinally, given their abundance of useful minerals and trace elements. Medicinal salt is often rich in minerals such as calcium, iron, bromide, and magnesium. Generally, every usage for salt in this chapter will work better with sea salt, as standard iodized table salt is often stripped of valuable minerals.

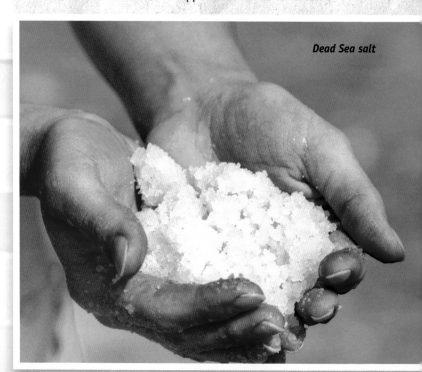

Dead Sea salt

Dead Sea salt is high in magnesium, calcium, and bromide. This variety of salt is well-known for its ability to help reduce joint pain and stress, as well as keeping skin looking younger by minimizing wrinkles. Some of the minerals found in unprocessed Dead Sea salt can be toxic when ingested, and so only Dead Sea salt that is specifically labeled as food-grade should be eaten or used in food.

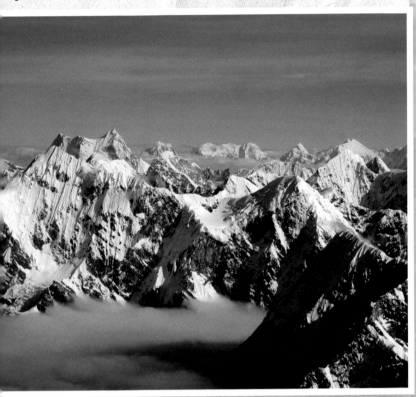

he Himalaya mountains

Himalayan crystal salt is famous for its high mineral count; it contains 84 minerals and trace elements such as copper, magnesium, and iron—the cause of Himalayan salt's characteristic pink hue. Himalayan salt is generally believed to provide more flavor to meals than regular table salt when used in cooking, and is commonly used in salt therapy to promote improved respiratory health.

Epsom salt is a naturally occurring compound of magnesium and sulfate, as opposed to the sodium chloride composition of most edible salts. As such, it should not be used in food or ingested without the express instruction of your doctor. Epsom salt is best known for its use as a muscle pain reliever, but it can also be used to help maintain healthy blood circulation and treat conditions like athlete's foot.

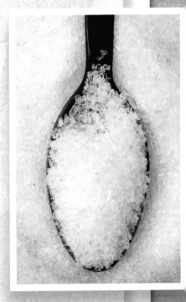

Epsom salt

43

WELLNESS

SOOTHE A SORE THROAT

Gargling salt water is one of the most reliable and commonly used methods of treating a sore throat. The salt helps flush out unwanted bacteria in your mouth and throat, while also acting as a painkiller by reducing inflammation.

Mix ½ tablespoon salt with 8 ounces water until dissolved. Gargle the salt water for several seconds before spitting it out.

Tip: Warm water may be more effective here, as salt will dissolve faster in warm water than in cold.

Tip 2: Especially coarse salt may irritate your throat if not completely dissolved, so finer grains of salt may be preferable here.

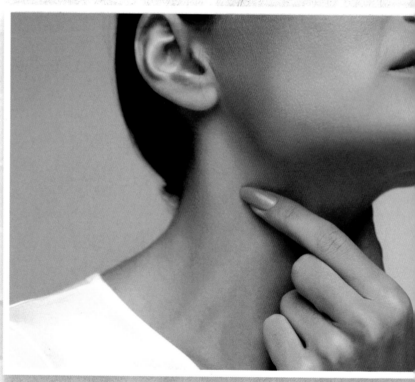

Helps aid a sore throat

SOOTHE SUNBURN

Epsom salt can be dissolved in water and sprayed or massaged onto a sunburn to reduce redness, pain, and itchiness. Mix a few tablespoons Epsom salt into a glass of warm water, and use either a spray bottle or a soft compress to coat the burned area with the solution.

WARNING!
Sunburned skin is sensitive, so you might not want to use coarse grained salt for this one.

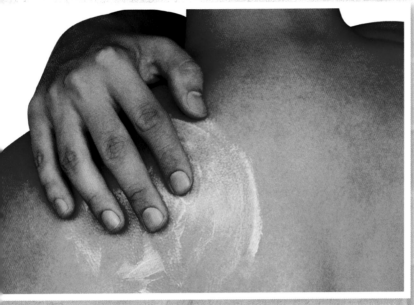

Soothe sunburn

TREAT CONGESTION, ALLERGIES, AND SINUS INFECTIONS

Because of its antibacterial and anti-inflammatory properties, salt can also be used to treat sinus infections and stuffy noses. The most effective way to use salt to treat congestion, inflammation, or a sinus infection is through a saltwater sinus rinse.

Mix ½ tablespoon salt with 8 ounces warm water in your neti pot until dissolved.

WARNING!
If using hot water, be sure to wait until the solution cools to room temperature before continuing.

Lean over a sink and tilt your head to one side, then slowly pour the saltwater solution into one nostril.

Make sure to breathe through your mouth, not your nose. Let gravity carry the solution through your nasal passage and out of your other nostril.

Gently blow your nose, then repeat the previous

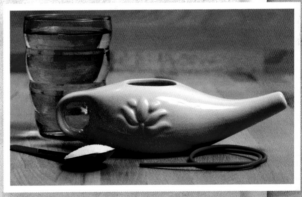

Neti pot

steps starting with your other nostril. Repeating this process daily will help you achieve the best results, but even one or two rinses should produce immediate relief.

How does this work? Rinsing your nasal passages with salt water rehydrates your sinus's mucous membranes, flushes away debris, and reduces inflammation; all of which make it easier to breathe through your nose.

WELLNESS

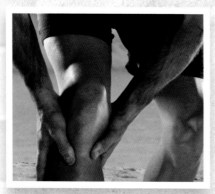

Treat muscle pain

RELIEVE MUSCLE AND JOINT PAIN
A saltwater bath is a great way to help relieve the pain and stiffness in aching joints and muscles. This can help soothe physical injuries, chronic pain, rheumatoid arthritis, or even simply sore feet after a long day of work. You can use sea salt or kosher salt, or exotic salts like Dead Sea or Himalayan salt for added health benefits and relaxation. Iodized table salt should generally be avoided when running a saltwater bath. To get the best results in terms of pain relief in muscles and joints, use Epsom salt or a mix of Epsom salt and another coarse salt of your choice.

Add two cups Epsom salt or another coarse salt of your choice to a full bathtub and soak for 15–45 minutes. If using a smaller or less full tub for just your feet and ankles, use ½ cup salt.

Tip: Try adding a few drops of essential oil and a little food coloring to make a DIY bath bomb, for added relaxation and stress relief.

BOMBS AWAY!
The following basic recipe makes 12 bombs, so be sure you've purchased enough molds to accommodate them. The batter hardens quickly, so you can't mold the bombs in smaller batches.

Fizzing Bath Bombs

- 4 ounces Epsom salts • 8 ounces baking soda • 4 ounces cornstarch
- 4 ounces citric acid • 2½ tablespoons coconut or olive oil
- 1 tablespoon water • 2 teaspoons essential oil, your choice
- 4–6 drops of food coloring • 12–18 silicon molds

In a large bowl mix the dry ingredients together so there are no clumps. Place the wet ingredients in a jar and shake them up. Then add the liquid to the dry ingredients in slow, tiny increments. This is really critical—you don't want the mixture to start fizzing prematurely if the baking soda starts reacting to the citric acid. Stop blending and wait if fizzing begins. The finished mixture

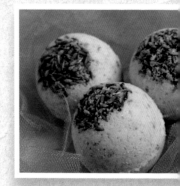

should just barely clump together. Now quickly press the mixture into the molds, because it will start to harden almost immediately. The bombs should take approximately one day to dry, a bit longer if your molds have intricate details. Test one bomb in the tub and watch it explode into colorful bubbles. Wrap each bomb in cellophane and prepare to hand them out, perhaps with a small tag describing their scent.

TREAT DEHYDRATION

Your body loses a lot of salt and water when you're sick or when you physically exert yourself. Whether you're recovering from a bout of food poisoning or you're an athlete coming to the end of some intense training, salt is vital to recovering a healthy balance of electrolytes in your body. For a drink to help you rehydrate quickly, dissolve 6 teaspoons sugar and ½ to 1 teaspoon salt in 4 cups water.

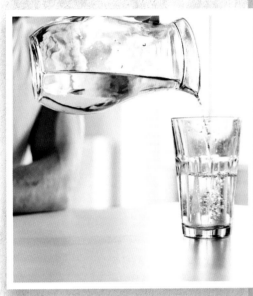

Rehydrate

TREAT INSECT BITES

If you've been stung or bitten by an insect, salt can help provide immediate relief. Soaking the infected area in salt water—Epsom salts will work especially well here—will help reduce pain, swelling, and itchiness caused by anything from a mosquito bite to a bee sting.

WARNING!
Take slow sips, especially if severely dehydrated, as drinking too fast may upset your stomach.

WARNING!
If you are allergic to the insect that bit or stung you, seek medical help immediately.

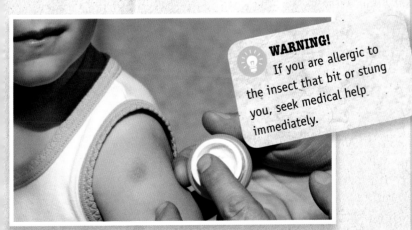

Treat insect bites

WELLNESS

SOOTHE POISON IVY

Soaking in salt water can help reduce inflammation and discomfort caused by allergic reactions to poison ivy and poison oak. This will not cure the symptoms of poison ivy exposure altogether, but it will soothe the affected area and rehydrate dry skin, helping reduce itchiness. Make sure to thoroughly wash off any poison ivy oil before taking a bath, to avoid spreading the rash to other parts of your body.

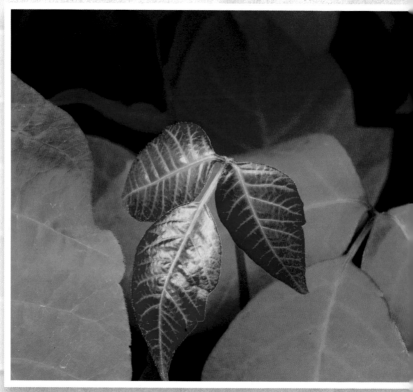

Poison ivy

COOL A BURNED TONGUE

To relieve some of the pain of a burned mouth or tongue—after eating something too hot, for example—mix ½ teaspoon salt with 8 ounces water and rinse your mouth out every hour or until the pain fades.

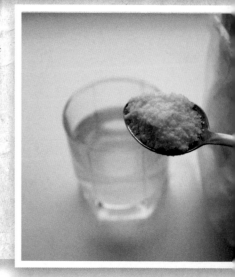

Ease a burned mouth or tongue

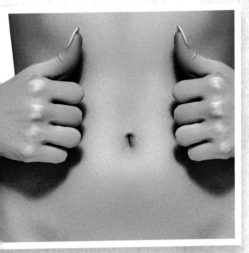
Aid healthy digestion

AID DIGESTION

Mix 1 tablespoon any food-grade salt of your choice with a glass of warm water at the beginning of every day. Drinking this solution on an empty stomach first thing in the morning will help kick-start your digestive system and metabolism for the rest of the day.

Tip: Try including some honey, ginger, or lemon in this morning drink to improve the flavor and help wake yourself up at the same time.

TREAT PUFFINESS AND SHADOWS UNDER EYES

To reduce the swelling and redness around your eyes that often occurs as a result of not enough (or low-quality) sleep, make a solution of sea salt and water and rinse the area around your eyes, nose, and upper cheeks. This should rejuvenate and diminish redness while also helping you refresh a little after a sleepless night.

Kick-start your day

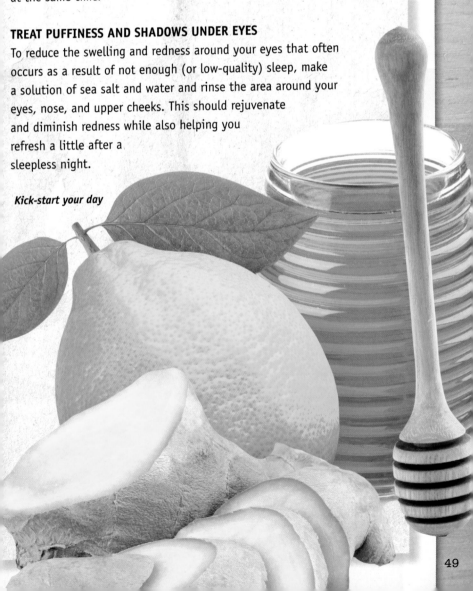

WELLNESS

SALT THERAPY (HALOTHERAPY)

Salt therapy, also known as halotherapy, is a centuries-old practice that revolves around the medical and therapeutic benefits of inhaling salt-infused air. While there are several ways to go about this, the most common method involves spending time in a room or cave in which the walls, floors, and ceiling are comprised almost entirely of salt. Originally, this was done by venturing into underground salt mines. In an attempt to modernize the practice of salt therapy, there are now locations all around the world where large quantities of Himalayan salt are imported and used to build specially-made salt therapy rooms. In some cases, high quality salt is ground down into miniscule, breathable particles and pumped into the air. Halotherapy is also occasionally performed by breathing in the steam produced by heating salt water.

The primary purpose of salt therapy is to improve respiratory health. Salt therapy claims to help alleviate the symptoms of allergies and asthma, as well as allowing for stress reduction through relaxation and meditation. It is thought that breathing in salt-saturated air for long

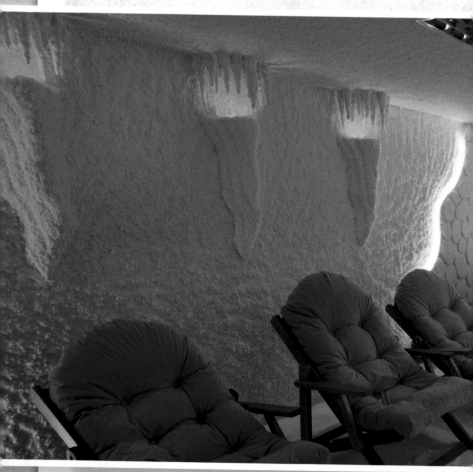

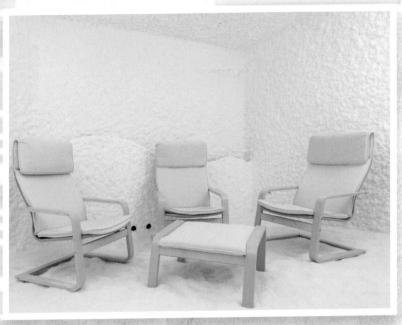

Cozy salt therapy room

periods of time helps reduce inflammation and mucus buildup in the lungs and throat, while also killing harmful bacteria that may otherwise irritate your airways.

Large salt therapy room

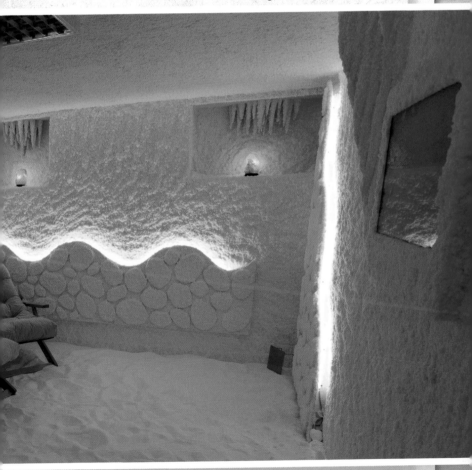

BEAUTY/PERSONAL

Salt has always been an excellent way to maintain the health of your body, but its uses go deeper than simply being a dietary requirement or a salve for injuries. Salt can also be used cosmetically, as a cost-effective exfoliant, face scrub, mouthwash, and more. The high mineral count in exotic salts like Himalayan sea salt is good for your skin and hair, and naturally coarse-grained salt is perfect for treating acne, softening skin, and treating dry or flaky lips.

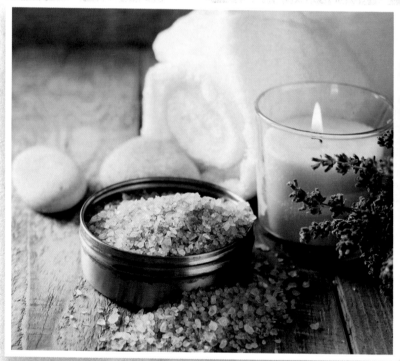

Colored bath salts

SOFTEN AND EXFOLIATE SKIN

Making a DIY salt scrub can be a cheap and effective way to soften and exfoliate your skin, while avoiding harsher ingredients that might irritate or dry out your skin.

Start by combining 1 cup sea salt with 1 tablespoon of either olive oil or coconut oil and mixing the two into a paste. Feel free to add a few drops of essential oil as well. Rub into your skin, then rinse.

Tip: For better skin rejuvenation and rehydration, add ¼ cup aloe vera gel to your salt scrub.

Tip 2: Store any unused salt scrub in an airtight container to keep it in good condition.

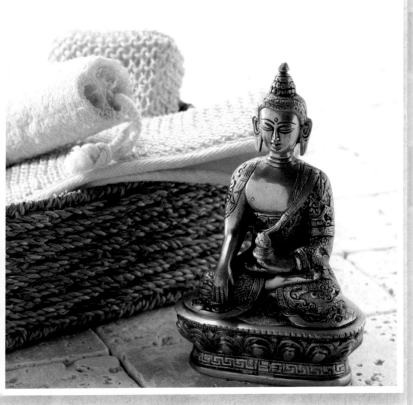

Use a salt scrub to exfoliate and relax

BRIGHTEN NAILS

If your nails are stained with dirt, ink, or nail polish, you can use a mixture of salt, lemon, and baking soda to return them to their former shine. Mix one teaspoon of each, apply the mixture to a soft cloth, and use the cloth to gently buff your nails until clean.

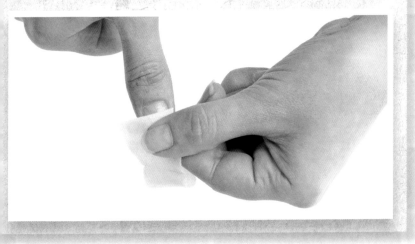

BEAUTY/PERSONAL

GET A CLOSER SHAVE

Use this exfoliating scrub in place of shaving cream to get a smoother, closer shave. Combine 1 tablespoon coarse sea (or kosher) salt, 1 cup unsused coffee grinds, and 2 tablespoons olive or coconut oil into a smooth paste, and scrub your skin vigorously. Shave off the paste for a smooth shave free of razor burn.

TREAT ACNE

Salt can be used to fight bouts of acne by killing bacteria, exfoliating your skin and pores, and reducing dryness and inflammation. The many essential minerals present in luxury salts like Himalayan crystal

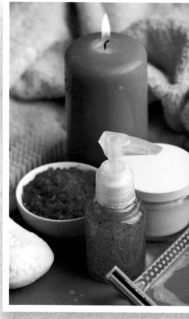

Shaving supplies

salt are also important, as they help promote healthy skin. There are quite a few ways to go about making a salt-based facial cleanser, so here are some of the most popular.

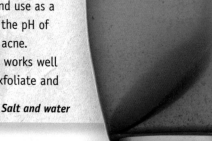

Salt combats acne

Salt and water is one of the simplest options, and should work well. Mix a few tablespoons salt with 1 cup water until completely dissolved. You can either massage this into your skin for a few minutes at a time, or spray it on yourself with a clean spray bottle.

For a more thorough cleanse, try combining 1 cup salt, 2 tablespoons grapefruit juice, 2 cups sugar, and 2–3 tablespoons coconut oil depending on consistency. Mix into a paste and use as a facial or body scrub to balance the pH of your skin, reduce oil, and fight acne.

Mixing honey with salt also works well to fight acne. The salt helps exfoliate and

Salt and water

open up clogged pores, and the honey acts as an antibiotic to fight the bacteria that causes acne. Stir together 2 tablespoons salt and 4 tablespoons honey, and apply as a paste to acne-affected areas. Leave on for a few minutes before rinsing thoroughly for best results.

EXFOLIATE DRY LIPS

To exfoliate and soften dry lips—with the added bonus of using a product that doesn't taste like soap if it ends up in your mouth—mix together ½ tablespoon sea salt and 1 tablespoon coconut oil into a paste and gently scrub your lips with it. For extra effect, include lime, lemon, or grapefruit juice (or zest) to the mixture. The end result should give you softer, smoother lips free of cracking and dry skin.

REDUCE DANDRUFF

Salt's ability to minimize oiliness in skin, exfoliate pores, and clean dry skin makes it perfect for treating dandruff. The simplest solution is to mix ½ tablespoon salt into your shampoo every time you wash your hair, massaging it into the roots to help exfoliate your scalp and prevent a buildup of dry skin. Be sure to rinse thoroughly afterwards to get rid of any lingering salt particles. If you have a little more time, you can also make your own dandruff-cleansing solution with sea salt, olive or coconut oil, and lemon juice. Mix together 2 tablespoons each, and massage it gently into your scalp for several minutes. Rinse thoroughly, then shampoo and condition as needed.

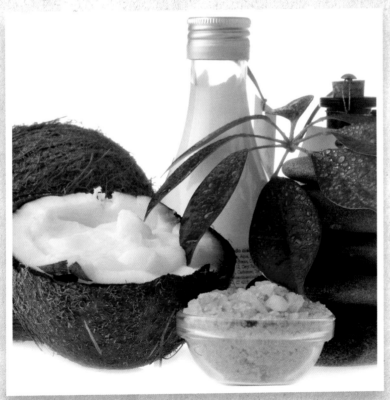

Dandruff-cleansing solution

BEAUTY/PERSONAL

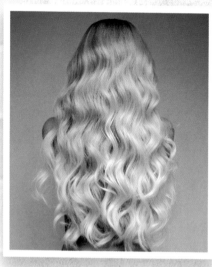

Create beach waves

CREATE TEXTURED, WAVY HAIR

Mix 1 teaspoon salt with 20 ounces warm water in a large spray bottle, and allow it to fully dissolve. Apply to towel-dried hair after a shower, and let your hair air-dry to give your hair a wavy, fresh-from-the-beach look.

WHITEN TEETH

To help whiten your teeth, use salt as an alternative to toothpaste. Simply dip your wet toothbrush in a pinch of fine sea salt and brush your teeth as you would normally. If you have sensitive teeth, or are worried that raw salt will damage your enamel, try dissolving a few tablespoons salt in warm water, dipping your brush in the solution, and brushing your teeth with that. Simply rinsing your mouth with saltwater will also help fight plaque, although with less dramatic results.

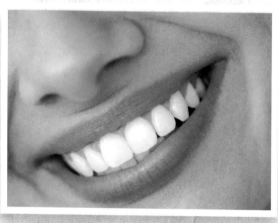

Have a beautiful smile

FRESHEN BREATH

A daily rinse with salt water will help improve your gum health, kill and flush out bacteria and food debris that cause bad breath, and fight any infections that might cause pain or inflammation. Dissolve a few tablespoons salt in a glass of warm water. Swish the solution in your mouth for a minute or two every morning.

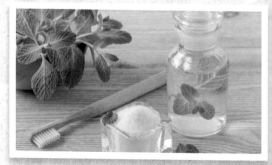

Helps to freshen breath

DIY SALT SCRUBS

You can use something as simple as a mixture of sea salt and coconut butter to make a soothing, exfoliating face and body scrub, but every recipe has room for improvement. Here are a few more natural, healthy body scrubs you can make in your own home, all of which will lead to brighter, softer skin, reducing your stress levels and revitalizing you for the rest of the day.

Salt-Banana Body Scrub

1 whole banana
3 tablespoons coarse Himalayan sea salt
¼ teaspoons essential oil of your choice

Mash ingredients together in a bowl or with a mortar and pestle until it forms a smooth paste, without actually grinding down the coarse salt itself. Scrub skin with a warm washcloth and rinse as usual.

Tomato Scrub

1 tomato with stem
Fine table salt, measured to preference

Cut off the top of the tomato and hold it by the stem. Pour some salt onto a plate, then dip the cut part of the tomato in the salt. Using a circular motion, buff your face with the salt-covered tomato. Keep dipping the tomato in salt to consistently exfoliate the skin.

Citrus "Wake-up" Scrub

½ cup coarse Himalayan sea salt
½ cup olive oil or coconut oil
1 teaspoon various citrus zest (mix lemon, orange, lime, and/or grapefruit)
Mix ingredients together into a smooth paste. During your morning shower, scrub onto skin and rinse with warm water.

Rejuvenating Lip Scrub

1 tablespoon powdered sugar
1 tablespoon fine table salt
1 teaspoon coconut or olive oil
1 tablespoon honey

Microwave honey in a microwave-safe container for about 20 seconds, then add other ingredients to form a paste. Rub onto lips with fingers, scrubbing to exfoliate. Let sit for about 2 minutes. Rinse with warm water. Save remainder in a glass container.
Tip: For more thorough exfoliation, you can gently apply this scrub to your lips with a soft-bristled toothbrush.

HOME

While salt is great for your health, it can also be extremely useful around the house. All the qualities that make salt such a good exfoliant and skin cleanser also help make it a powerful and natural all-purpose cleaning agent. You can use it raw to soak up grease or dyes from resistant stains, or use coarse sea salt as a scouring agent in soaps or cleansers to help scrub away food residue, rust, and all other kinds of accumulated debris. For delicate fabrics or surfaces that might be damaged by more abrasive salt, you might want to use fine grain or table salt.

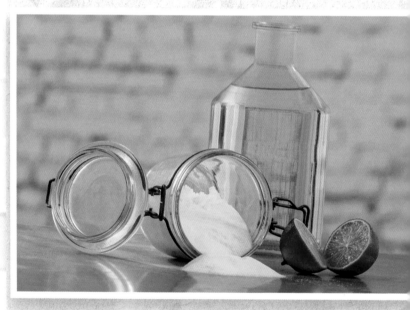

Salt, water, and lime

CLEAN STAINED CLOTHES
Bloodstains

Salt and water is an efficient and cost-effective way to remove bloodstains from clothes and other fabric. You can either rub dry salt into the stain first and then soak the garment in cold water, or you can simply soak the whole thing in a salt water bath. Follow up with a soap and water wash, and finally rinse with warm—not hot—water.
Tip: Don't use hot water, as that may result in the stain setting in deeper rather than washing out.

Tip 2: Using soda water instead of tap water can be even more effective, if available.

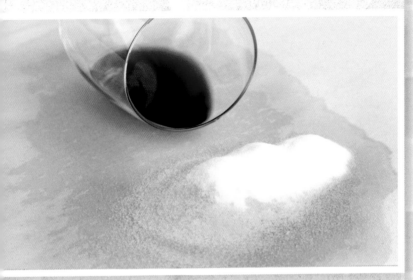

Fix a stain with salt

Wine stains

To remove red wine stains from your clothes, it's best to start as soon as possible after spilling the wine, so that the stain hasn't had time to dry and set. Blot the stain dry as much as you can without rubbing the wine further into the fabric. Then cover the stain with salt, allowing it to break up the stain and absorb as much of it as possible. Let it sit for a few minutes, then wash the garment with soap and warm water.

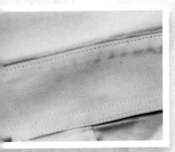

Clean grime and sweat

Sweat stains

To wash sweat stains or yellowing out of clothes, soak the fabric for several minutes in a solution of 4 tablespoons salt for every 1 quart of hot water. Let soak for several minutes and then wash as you otherwise would, and all the discoloration should vanish.

CLEAN AN IRON

Lay down a layer of salt on a heat-proof surface, heat iron to medium heat, and iron over the layer of salt. This should remove any rust, stains, or other residue on the metal. Make sure to wipe the iron clean before using it.

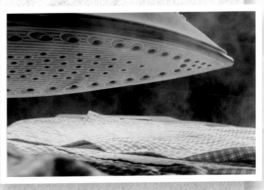

Clean the bottom of your iron

HOME

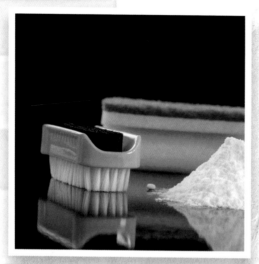

Use salt to scour pots and pans

CLEAN POTS AND PANS

To clean greasy or food-stained pans, use a mixture of salt and vinegar to scour away any unwanted debris. Pour salt and white vinegar into the pan, and swish around until the food and grease come loose. Rinse the pan and clean as normal.
Tip: Use a rough sponge to help scrub away any hard-to-clean food residue.

CLEAN UP RAW EGG

If you spill a raw egg on the floor or kitchen counter while cooking, you can use salt to make the cleanup a little easier. Pouring salt on the egg before you wipe it up makes the egg coagulate, making the job easier and less messy.

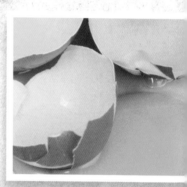

Clean egg spill

SMOTHER A GREASE FIRE

A grease fire is dangerous, and should never be put out with water. Pour a large amount of salt on a grease fire to safely smother the fire.

WARNING!
Never attempt to use water to smother a grease fire as this can cause an explosion

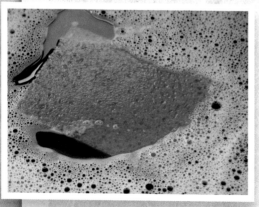

Soak a sponge in salt water

WASH A DIRTY SPONGE

You can naturally extend the life of a worn or dirty sponge by cleaning it with saltwater. Mix ¼ cup salt in 2 cups warm water, and soak your sponge in it for several hours. Once you remove it from the water and wring it dry, it should be perfectly clean again and ready for use.

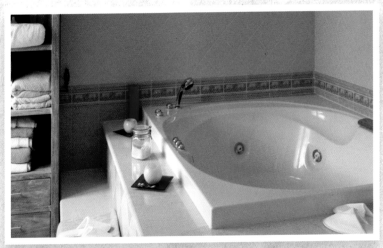

Clean a ceramic bathtub

CLEAN A STAINED BATHTUB

Salt can be used as an inexpensive cleaner to scrub stains out of the bathtub. Mix equal parts salt and turpentine to form a paste, then scrub stains from tub using a washcloth or a firm sponge. The stains will lift quickly and easily. Make sure to rinse your tub thoroughly before using it again.

UNCLOG A DRAIN

If your kitchen sink is clogged with food residue, this mixture of salt, baking soda, and vinegar makes a surprisingly effective drain cleaner. Pour ¼ cup baking soda and ¼ cup salt into a clogged drain, followed by ½ cup white vinegar. Let sit for about 20 minutes, then follow with a pot of boiling water. If the drain isn't completely cleared after this, repeating the process should produce the desired effects.

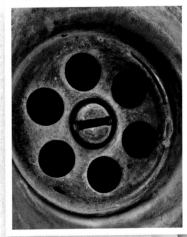

Use salt to unclog a drain

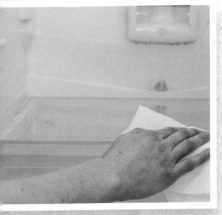

CLEAN A REFRIGERATOR

To clean your refrigerator's shelves and drawers after emptying it out—or to clean up after a spill—you can use a mixture of salt and selzer water as a refrigerator cleaner. The coarse texture of the salt will help scrub off any food residue or stubborn stains, as well as deodorizing your fridge for future use.

Clean your refrigerator

HOME

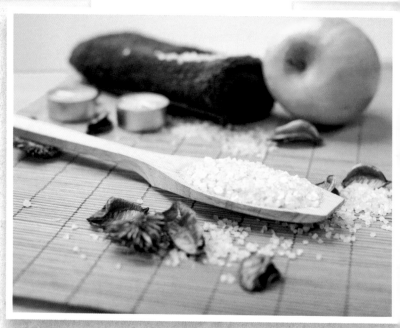

Use salt as a preservative

PREVENT FRUIT FROM BROWNING

Salt acts as a kind of natural preservative for everything from meat to fruits and vegetables. You can use salt water to extend the life of any apples and pears left unfinished, which is helpful if you frequently find yourself leaving fruit uneaten long enough that it starts to turn brown. Soak any piece of fruit in a saltwater solution for a few minutes, rinse and dry it off thoroughly—you probably don't want salty-tasting fruit— and it should last quite a bit longer before it starts to turn brown.

CLEAN OVEN SPILLS

Salt is great for soaking up grease from stains and loosening accumulated grime on kitchen surfaces. This combined with its abrasive nature makes it a great choice when cleaning tougher things such as stovetops or ovens. Start by applying a damp cloth to the area in question, then pour a liberal amount of salt wherever you can see stains. Leave it

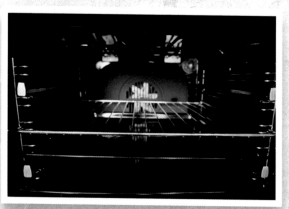

Clean an oven

there for several minutes to clump up the mess and make it easier to clean, and then wipe the area down with another damp cloth or sponge.

ANT BARRIER

One way to help deal with an ant problem—without setting down traps or poison that could be harmful to pets or small children around the house—is to line doorways and windowsills with salt. Sprinkle a line of salt anywhere you suspect ants or other insects may be entering your house, and you should see a noticeable decrease in the number of ants entering your home.

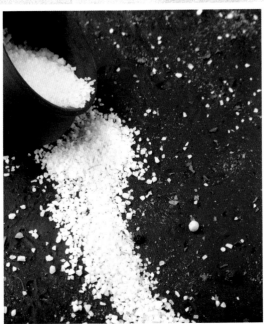

Keep insects out

PRESERVE CUT FLOWERS

To make cut flowers live a little longer before wilting or losing their color, mix about ½ teaspoon salt into the water in the vase. The salt should help keep the flowers colorful and lively for at least a few days longer than usual.

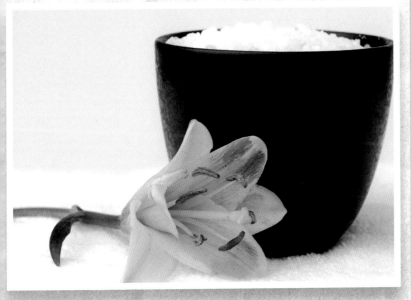

Keep flowers fresh

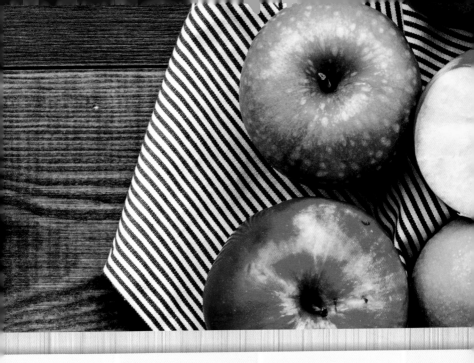

CHAPTER 3
VINEGAR

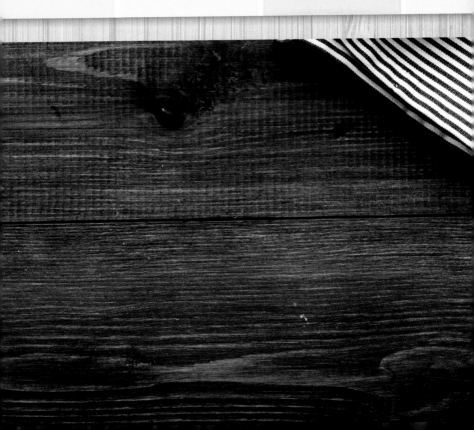

VINEGAR USES

Vinegar has dramatically increased in popularity as a pantry staple with wide-ranging benefits.

Made from apple juice, apple cider vinegar is a fermented liquid that can contain probiotics, or bacteria that help keep your digestive system healthy. Specifically, raw, unpasteurized apple cider vinegar is the most beneficial for your gut. It also has a variety of benefits that can improve your health and beauty routine.

While apple cider vinegar has a variety of health and beauty benefits, distilled white vinegar is an incredibly versatile pantry staple. It is excellent for cleaning around the home and can be incorporated easily into your daily routine.

1

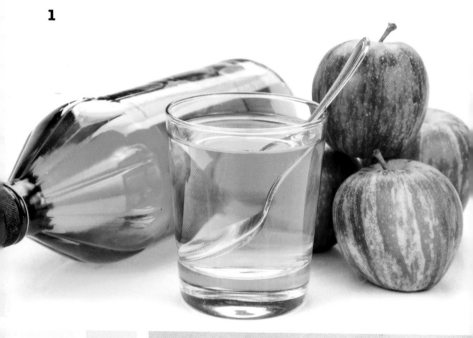

1 Apple cider
  vinegar in a
  glass
2 Types of vinegar
3 Vinegar with
  baking soda
4 Raw,
  unpasteurized
  apple cider
  vinegar

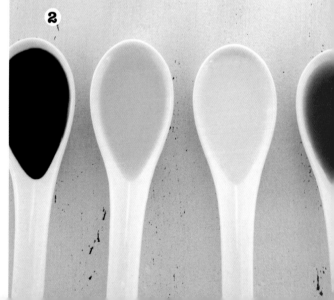

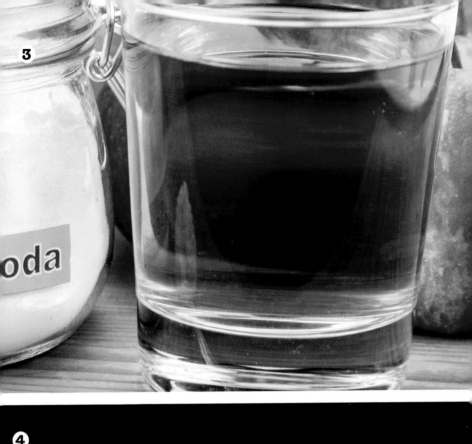

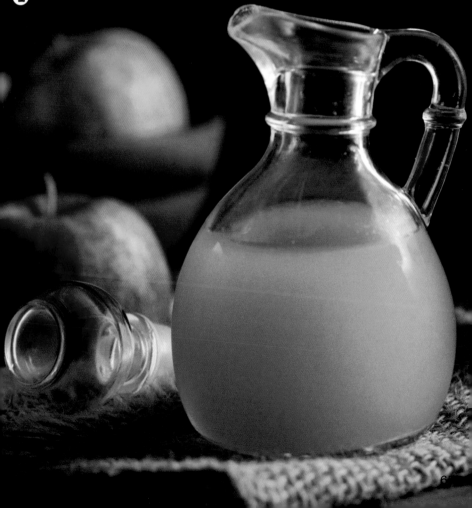

WELLNESS

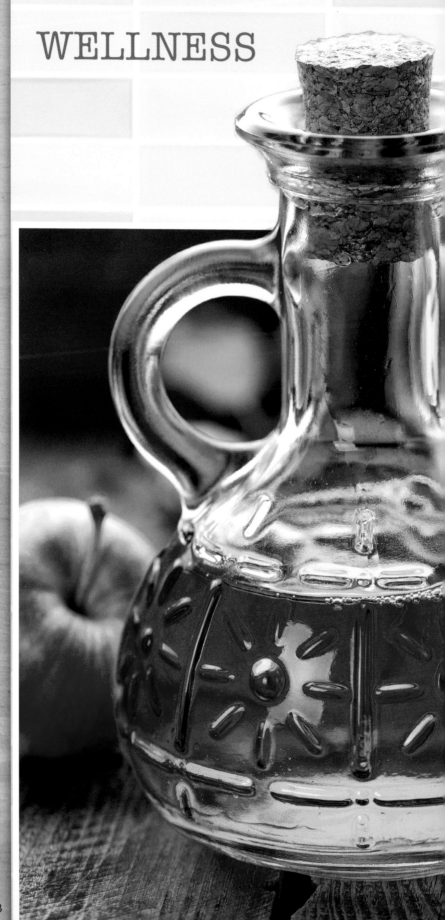

The bacteria in raw, unpasteurized apple cider vinegar has been proven to be very beneficial for your gut and digestive system health. Apple cider vinegar (ACV) has antifungal properties and is therefore an effective way to combat foot odor or work as a natural mouthwash. From alleviating cold symptoms to helping with weight loss, apple cider vinegar is incredibly versatile in the ways it can improve your health and home.

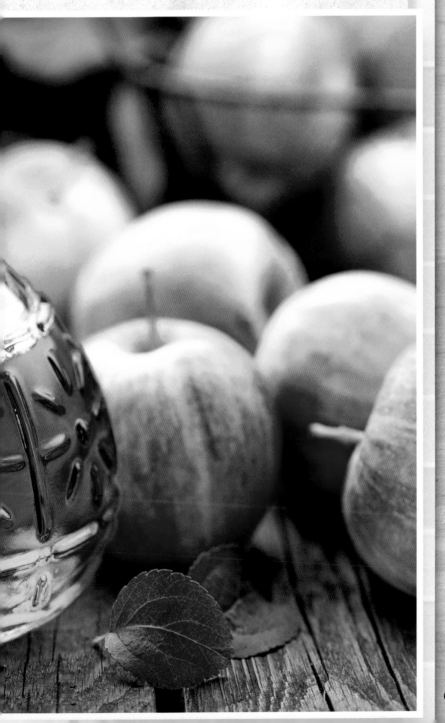

WELLNESS

REDUCE ACID REFLUX

Many times, acid reflux and heartburn are caused by the underproduction of stomach acid, rather than too much. The acidity of ACV mimics the environment of the stomach and can counter the painful symptoms of reflux or heartburn. One teaspoon of ACV may eliminate those symptoms.

To prevent acid reflux, add 1 teaspoon honey and 1 teaspoon ACV to a glass of warm water and drink 30 minutes before you eat.

RELIEVE IRRITATED SKIN

Add 1 cup ACV to your bathwater to soothe sunburned skin. For a less general method, mix a 1:3 ratio of ACV to water and apply a cloth soaked in the mixture directly to the irritated skin.

For bug bites, apply a 1:1 mixture of ACV and water directly to the bite using a soaked cloth. You can also soak the affected area in the mixture.

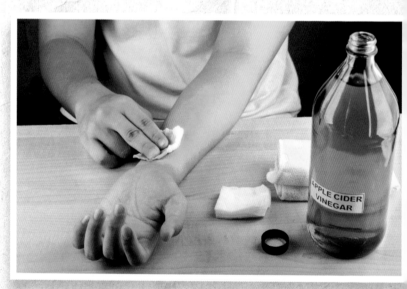

Use apple cider vinegar for bug bites

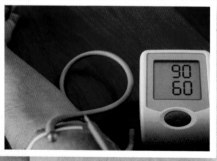

ACV may help to lower blood pressure

LOWER BLOOD PRESSURE

Some studies suggest that the acetic acid in ACV may help to lower blood pressure. Be sure to talk to your doctor before starting any treatment plan involving ACV.

WARNING! ACV should never ingested undiluted.

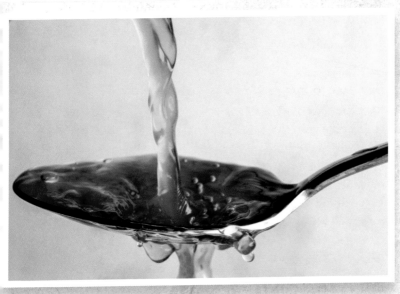

Raw, unfiltered apple cider vinegar

KILL FUNGUS

To eliminate and prevent toe or foot fungus, soak your feet in 1 cup ACV and warm water. For skin fungus or yeast, apply a 1:3 mixture of ACV and water to the area.

Tip: If you have sensitive skin, do a patch test before soaking your skin. If the vinegar mixture is too harsh, dilute it further by adding water.

SOOTHE A SORE THROAT

ACV has antibacterial properties, so it can be very helpful in combating a sore throat. Mix ¼ cup ACV and ¼ cup warm water and gargle every hour or so to nip a sore throat in the bud.

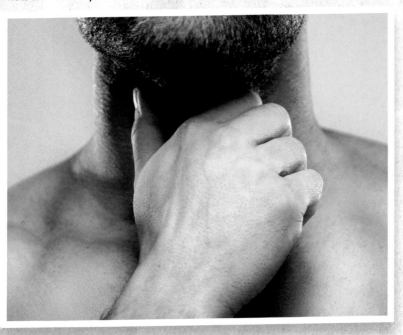

Drink diluted apple cider vinegar for a sore throat

WELLNESS

WEIGHT LOSS

The acetic acid in ACV can suppress your appetite, boost your metabolism, and reduce water retention. Taking 1–2 teaspoons ACV in water daily can give you the helping hand to lose some extra weight.

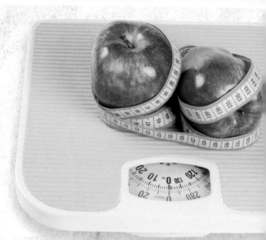

ACV can promote weight loss

ENERGY BOOST

The amino acids in ACV can counteract lactic acid build up in the body, which is often a result of exercise or extreme stress and leads to fatigue. By adding 1 tablespoon ACV to 8 ounces water, you can counteract the fatigue and give yourself an energy boost.

ELIMINATE CRAMPS

Leg cramps are often caused by low potassium levels and/or dehydration. Combat both possible culprits by drinking 2 teaspoons ACV and 1 teaspoon honey in 8 ounces warm water whenever you experience muscle cramps.

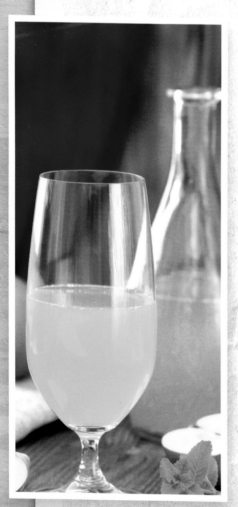

Diluted ACV for energy

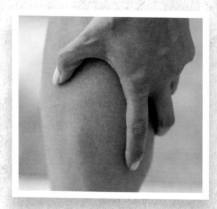

ACV can help with cramps

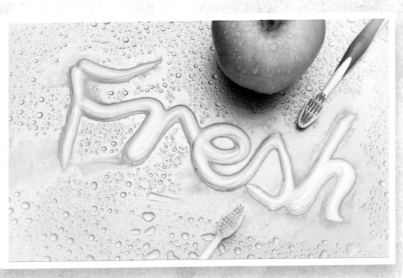

Gargle ACV for bad breath

KILL BAD BREATH

If you have persistent bad breath, try gargling with a 1:1 solution of ACV and water. The antibacterial properties of ACV will help kill the germs that cause bad breath without the harsh effects of a mouthwash that contains alcohol.

DETOX WITH ACV

Apple cider vinegar has been used for detoxification and health benefits for thousands of years. Raw, unfiltered apple cider vinegar contains good bacteria that is highly beneficial for the gut and intestines, as well as various minerals, vitamins, and enzymes. There are a variety of benefits that can result from consuming an apple cider vinegar drink daily, including helping with weight control, giving the body a dose of enzymes, aiding with healthy digestion, supporting a healthy immune system, increasing potassium intake, and adding good bacteria for improved gut and immune function. There are many variations on an apple cider vinegar detox, so no matter your flavor preferences, there will be a delicious option available.

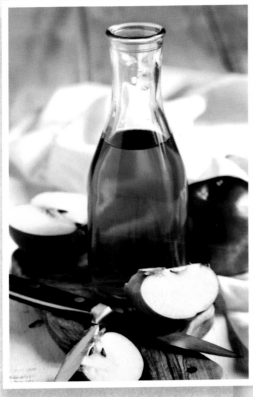

Make a detox drink with ACV

WELLNESS

Simple ACV Detox

2 tablespoons ACV

1 cup warm water

1 tablespoon sweetener (honey, maple syrup, etc.)

Combine ingredients in a glass and stir thoroughly. For best results, add the sweetener and ACV to warm water to enable the sweetener to dissolve.

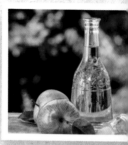

ACV from fresh apples

Classic Lemon Water ACV

1 cup water

1 tablespoon ACV

1 tablespoon lemon juice

½ teaspoon cinnamon, ground

1 pinch cayenne pepper (optional)

Honey to taste (optional)

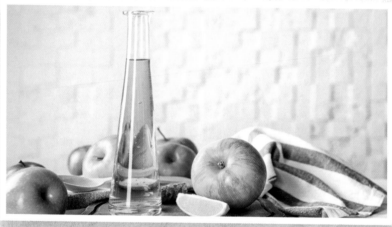

Create a detox drink

Cranberry Juice Detox

1 tablespoon ACV

¾ cup water

½ cup cranberry juice

Splash lime juice (optional)

Cranberries contain high quantity and quality antioxidants, which can prevent cell damage caused by oxidative stress. Cranberries also have anti-inflammatory properties that are amplified when combined with ACV.

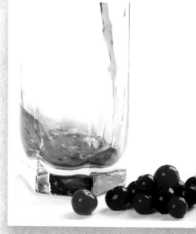

Add cranberries to your detox drink

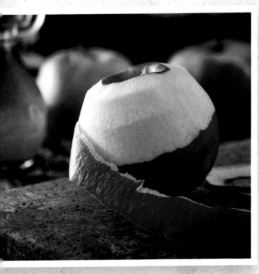

Detox Smoothie

1 tablespoon ACV
¼ cup water
1 cup apple, peeled
and sliced
2 tablespoons avocado
¼ cup ice

*Blend all ingredients
until smooth and serve
chilled*

Green Tea Detox

1 cup green tea or mint tea
1 tablespoon ACV
Honey to taste
Mint to taste

Prepare green tea (or mint tea, if desired) and add honey and ACV.

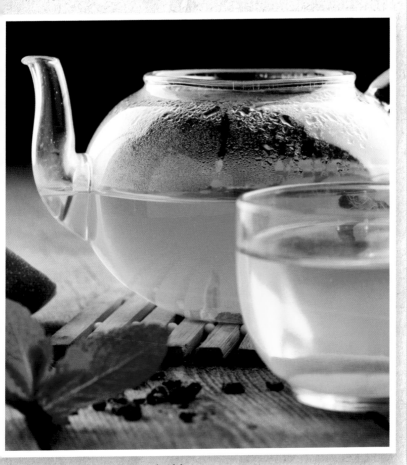

Green tea is excellent for your health

WELLNESS

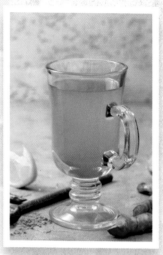

ACV detox drink

Want the benefits of the classic Lemon Water ACV detox drink in a sweeter drink? Try this Lemon & Cayenne Pepper detox.

Lemon & Cayenne Detox

1 cup water
1 tablespoon ACV
1 tablespoon lemon juice
1 teaspoon cayenne pepper
1 teaspoon honey

In a glass, combine all ingredients. Use warm water for best results and stir thoroughly.

Hot ACV Detox

2 cinnamon sticks
4 cloves
1½ cup water
2 tablespoons ACV
2 tablespoons honey
Lemon slices (optional)

Bring cinnamon, cloves, and water to a boil. Remove from heat and let cool, then add ACV, honey, and a slice of lemon if desired.

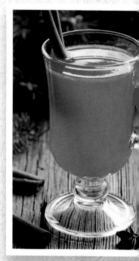

Warm ACV drink for cold day

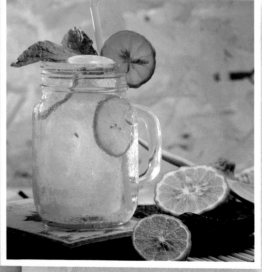

Cool ACV limeade

ACV Limeade

1 cup water
2 tablespoons ACV
½ cup limeade

To make your limeade, combine 1 cup fresh squeezed lime juice and 1 cup granulated sugar in a large pitcher and stir. Add 1½–2 quarts water (to taste) and stir well. Serve over ice and garnish with lime slices and mint sprigs.

Very Berry Smoothie Detox

1 cup fresh or frozen mixed berries
1 banana
1 cup almond, coconut, or cashew milk
1 teaspoon vanilla extract
2 tablespoons ACV
Pinch of salt

Combine all ingredients and blend until smooth.

Apple ACV Detox Drink

2 tablespoons ACV
2 tablespoons organic apple juice
1 cup water
4 drops vanilla extract
Pinch of cinnamon
½ teaspoon sugar (optional)

Mix all ingredients and serve over ice.

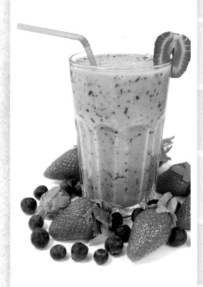

ACV detox smoothie

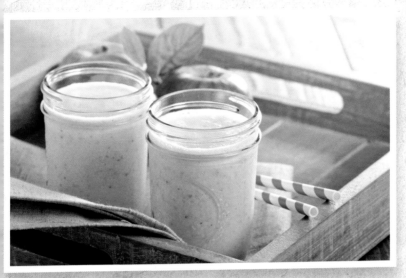

Apple cinnamon smoothie

Apple Pie ACV Detox Smoothie

1 apple, peeled and sliced
1 banana
1½ cups water
1 teaspoon cinnamon
½ teaspoon vanilla extract
3 ice cubes

Combine all ingredients and blend until smooth.

WELLNESS

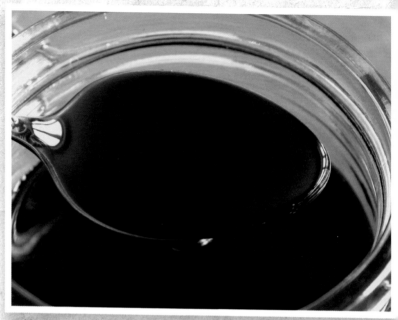

Add molasses with water and ACV for an uplifting detox drink

Molasses ACV Detox

1½ cups water
2 tablespoons ACV
2 tablespoons blackstrap molasses

In a glass, combine all ingredients and stir well.

Strawberry Blueberry ACV Smoothie

¼ cup blueberries
3 large strawberries
1 banana
¼ cup water
¼ cup chia seeds
1 tablespoon ACV
3 ice cubes
Mint leaves (optional)

Combine all ingredients (except mint leaves) and blend until smooth. Garnish with mint leaves if desired.

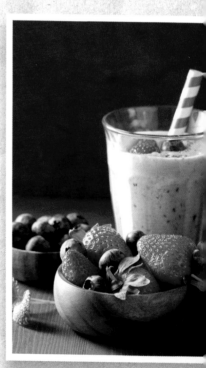

Berries in an ACV smoothie

Pink Drink ACV Detox

1 cup grapefruit juice
2 tablespoons ACV
1 tablespoon honey

In a glass, combine all ingredients and stir well.

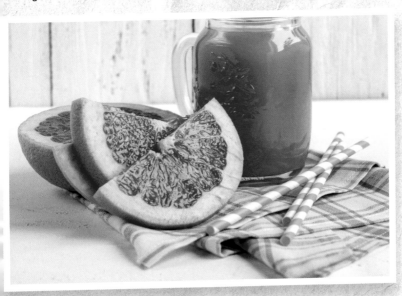

Grapefruit juice and ACV

Blueberry ACV Detox

2 tablespoons fresh blueberries
1 tablespoon ACV
2 tablespoons lemon juice
2 teaspoons maple syrup
1 cup water
Mint leaves (optional)

Mix all ingredients into a glass and stir.
Add ice and mint if desired.

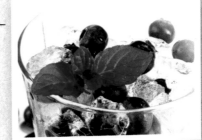

Garnish with mint leaves

Tip: *Crush blueberries with the back of a spoon in your drink to release the flavor.*

Cranberry-Orange Detox

¼ cup cranberry juice
¼ cup orange juice
¾ cup water
2 tablespoons ACV

In a glass, combine all ingredients and stir well.

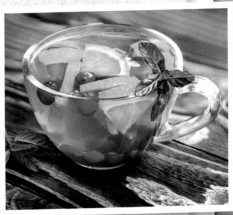

Cranberries with orange juice

BEAUTY/PERSONAL

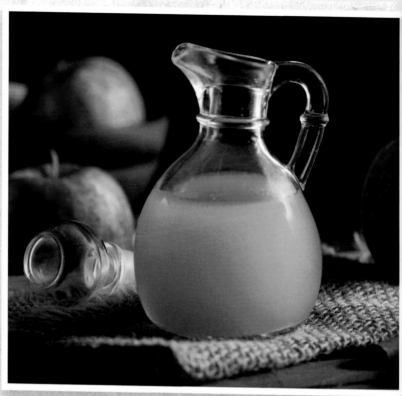

Add apple cider vinegar into your beauty routine

Apple cider vinegar has been proven to be beneficial for your skin and hair, being a natural way to beat dandruff and help eliminate acne. Apple cider vinegar contains high levels in acetic, citric, and malic acids as well as vitamins, enzymes, mineral salts, and amino acids; all of which are beneficial for your gut and skin. Additionally, apple cider vinegar's antibacterial, antiviral, anti-inflammatory, and antifungal properties make it an excellent choice for combating acne, oily hair, stained teeth, and irritated skin. Try adding apple cider vinegar into your beauty routine for a healthy solution to any beauty problems you've been facing.

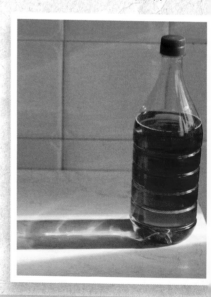

NATURAL TONER
ACV is an excellent natural toner that firms the skin

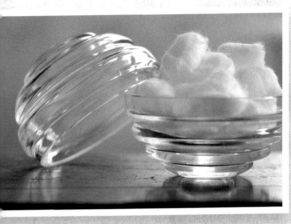

without drying it. The antibacterial properties of ACV can help keep acne under control, while the malic and lactic acids found in ACV can soften and exfoliate skin, reduce the appearance of redness, and maintain a healthy pH balance of your skin. Mix 1 tablespoon ACV with 2 cups water, and use a cotton pad or round to apply the mixture to your face to tighten your skin. There is no need to rinse, as the vinegar smell will dissipate once it dries. If the mixture is too harsh, dilute it further by adding water. This ACV toner will stimulate circulation and minimize the visibility of pores, while the antiseptic and antibacterial properties can prevent breakouts. This method is particularly beneficial for people with oily skin, as ACV has astringent properties that causes the skin to contract.

Tip: Store your ACV mixture in the fridge for an extra cooling effect.

HEALTHY HAIR RINSE

Create a mixture of 2 tablespoons ACV with 1 cup water. Store this mixture in a bottle to keep next to your shampoo of choice. After washing your hair in your usual method, tilt your head back and rinse your hair with your ACV mixture, making sure to avoid your eyes. Rinse thoroughly and condition your hair as usual. Any vinegar smell will dissipate once your hair dries. The acetic acid in ACV can help remove any buildup or residue from your hair products and keep your hair shiny.

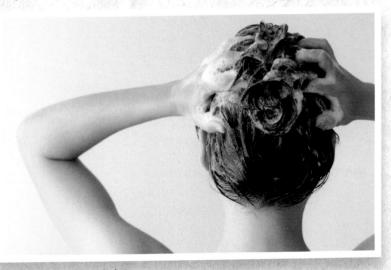

Use ACV to clean your hair

BEAUTY/PERSONAL

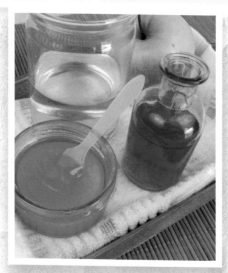

ELIMINATE RAZOR RASH
The anti-inflammatory properties of ACV can soothe irritated skin while the acetic acid can soften skin to alleviate ingrown hair growth. Use a cotton ball or round to apply undiluted ACV to the skin.

Tip: Try applying a light layer of honey to your skin first and rinse after 5 minutes before applying the ACV.

Use ACV and honey to minimize razor rash

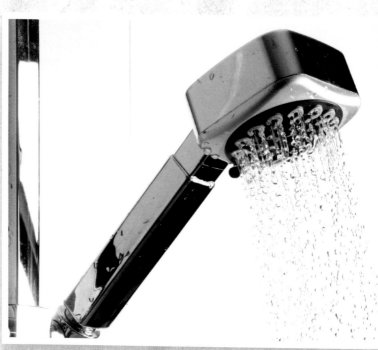

Use ACV in the shower

ELIMINATE DANDRUFF
To treat dandruff, create a mixture of equal parts ACV and water in a spray bottle. Before showering, spray your roots liberally with this mixture and let it sit for at least 15 minutes. Massage your scalp vigorously before showering, then wash your hair normally to help prevent and eliminate dandruff naturally. For best results, repeat the process 1–2 times per week.

Tip: Avoid getting the ACV mixture in your eyes.

NO MORE STINKY FEET

In a shallow basin, combine 1 cup ACV with 4 cups water. Soak your feet for 15 to 30 minutes, then rinse and dry your feet. The antimicrobial properties of ACV help deodorize your feet, while the antifungal properties can help combat and prevent fungal conditions such as athlete's foot.

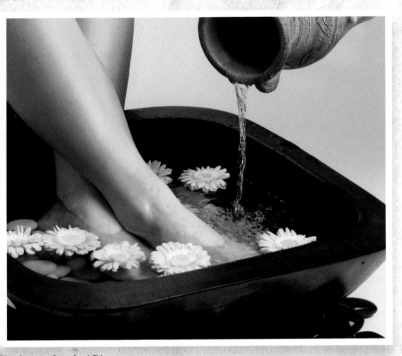

Soak your feet in ACV

WHITEN TEETH

If you want to naturally whiten your teeth, try gargling with ACV in the morning. Vinegar can help to remove stains, whiten teeth, and kill bacteria in your mouth and gums. Make a mixture of 1 part ACV to 3 parts water and use as mouthwash twice daily to help eliminate stains.

The acidic nature of ACV can help reduce any yellow staining on your teeth. Discoloration can occur due to drinking coffee, tea, or red wine; using tobacco products; and other factors.

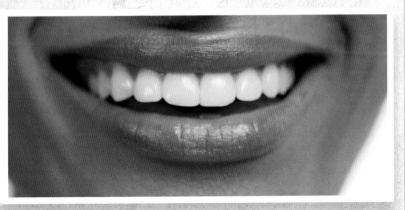

Use ACV to whiten teeth

HOME

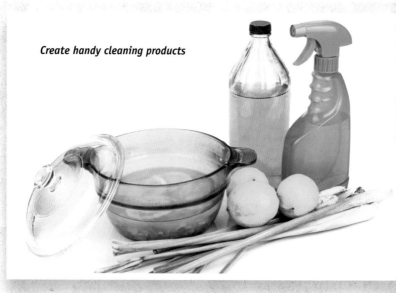

Create handy cleaning products

Many commercial cleaning agents commonly used around the house contain chemicals that are harmful for your health, the health of your children and pets, and the environment. Vinegar, particularly distilled white vinegar, is an incredibly versatile cleaning agent that can be used on anything from shower heads to countertops to microwaves. Distilled white vinegar is very inexpensive, natural, and nontoxic, making it environmentally safe and family-friendly. Its acidity and natural disinfectant properties makes it the natural go-to for combating grease, grime, and mineral deposits. Whether used alone or in combination with other pantry staples, vinegar is a natural cleaning wonder.

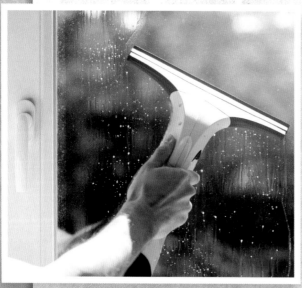

Use vinegar to clean your windows

WINDOW CLEANER

To thoroughly clean your windows without using harsh chemicals, make a mixture of equal parts distilled white vinegar and water. Spray your windows or apply with a sponge and wipe clean.

Tip: If you're using a squeegee to dry your windows, wet the blade before you use it so it won't skip.

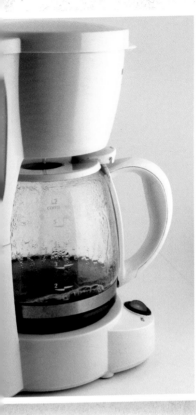

COFFEE MAKER CLEANSE

Fill the reservoir of your coffee maker with distilled white vinegar and run it through a brewing cycle to dissolve any old coffee buildup and stains. Once the cycle is complete, empty the carafe and run another full brewing cycle with just water.

FURNITURE POLISH

To add a sheen to your wooden furniture, make your own polish using vinegar. Combine ¼ cup white vinegar with 1 cup olive oil to clean and condition wood furniture. You can add a few drops of lemon or orange oil for a deodorizing effect.

Clean your coffee maker

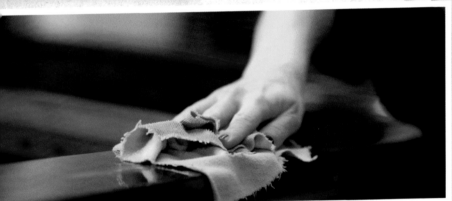

DIY wood polish

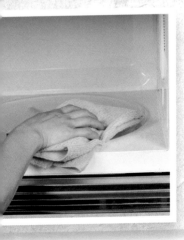

CLEAN YOUR MICROWAVE

If you have food buildup in your microwave, try this method. In a bowl, combine ¼ cup white vinegar and 1 cup water. Place in the microwave and turn the microwave on until steam forms on the window. Then, after waiting for it to cool, remove the bowl and give the inside of your microwave a wipe; the residue should come straight off.

HOME

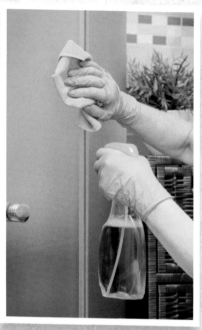

Use a spray bottle to clean your shower

MAINTAIN SHOWER DOORS

To prevent soap scum buildup on your shower doors or walls, wipe the clean surfaces with a sponge or rag soaked in white vinegar and let dry. Do not rinse or buff the vinegar away.

FLOWER FOOD

You can keep your cut flowers fresh much longer by adding 2 tablespoons white vinegar and 2 tablespoons sugar to the water in a 1 quart vase. Trim 1 inch off the ends of your flowers every few days and change the water regularly to promote longevity.

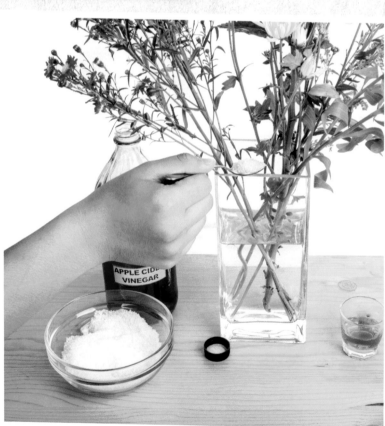

Feed your flowers with vinegar

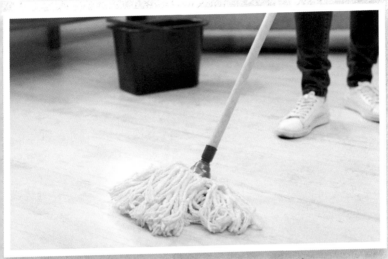

Mop using vinegar

FLOOR CLEANER

For an effective floor cleaner that won't harm your pets or children, combine ½ cup white vinegar with ½ gallon warm water. This method is safe on tile and wooden floors alike.

Tip: Undiluted vinegar is acidic, so be sure to test this mixture on your floors in an unobtrusive place before use.

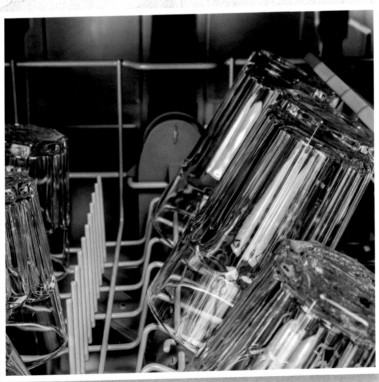

Eliminate spots on glassware

SPARKLING GLASSES

Add 1½ to 2 cups white vinegar to the bottom of your dishwasher for sparklingly clean glassware and dishes. Run your dishwasher on its regular cycle with your usual detergent.

HOME

COUNTERTOPS

Make a mixture of equal parts white vinegar and water to easily clean your countertops. Simply spray or wipe the mixture onto the surface using a rag or sponge and clean normally.

Tip: While vinegar is safe for most surfaces, avoid cleaning countertops that are granite, marble, and soapstone as it can cause pitting.

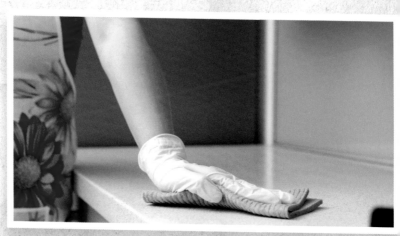

Wipe countertops with vinegar

REMOVE TARNISH

To remove tarnish from your copper, brass, and pewter cutlery or kitchenware, make a paste with 1 teaspoon salt, ½ cup white vinegar, and ½ teaspoon flour. Apply this mixture to the metal and let it sit for 15 minutes. Rinse with water and polish with a soft, dry cloth.

Tip: Avoid using paper towels to polish your metalware, as they can scratch the surface.

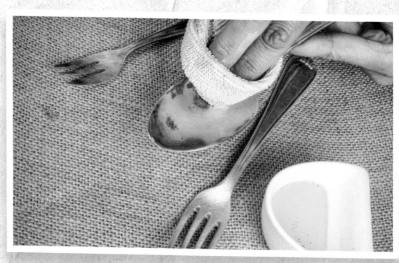

Polish silverware

CLOGGED SHOWERHEAD

Mineral build-up in showerheads can occur over time, especially if the water in your area is hard. This buildup affects the water pressure and overall quality of your shower. To dissolve this buildup, fill a small plastic bag with white vinegar and position the bag so the shower head sits in the vinegar. Use a rubber band or zip tie to hold the bag in place and let it sit overnight. Once you have removed the bag, run your shower to remove any buildup or remaining vinegar.

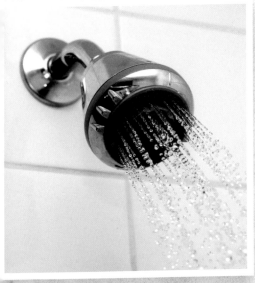

Regain good water pressure

FABRIC SOFTENER

Add 1 cup white vinegar to your laundry during the final wash cycle to soften clothes and remove static cling. It's a cheap way to get soft, clean clothes while helping to protect the environment.

CLEAN YOUR TUB

Remove any film that develops in your tub by using baking soda and vinegar. Spray or wipe the surfaces of your tub with white vinegar and then sprinkle baking soda over the same area. Rinse away with clean water.

For more stubborn grime, let the vinegar and baking soda sit for a few minutes, or add some elbow grease and buff the spot with a bristle brush or damp sponge.

Tip: Fiberglass tubs and showers are likely to scratch, so be sure to only use a sponge.

CUTTING BOARDS

To clean and sanitize your cutting boards, simply spray the surface with undiluted white vinegar, wipe, and rinse clean.

Tip: For wooden cutting boards that will last a long time, follow up with mineral oil or a cutting-board-specific wood oil to seal and protect the wood.

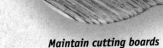

Maintain cutting boards

PET CARE

Pets are such important part of our lives and when they are suffering from itchy ears or skin, you'll want to help. Apple cider vinegar can be used to effectively remedy a number of complaints your cat or dog may be suffering from. Organic, raw, unfiltered apple cider vinegar will be most effective to relieve itchy skin, dirty ears, and keep away pests such as fleas and ticks. If you have concerns for your pet's health, give apple cider vinegar a try, but be sure to talk to a veterinarian if problems persist.

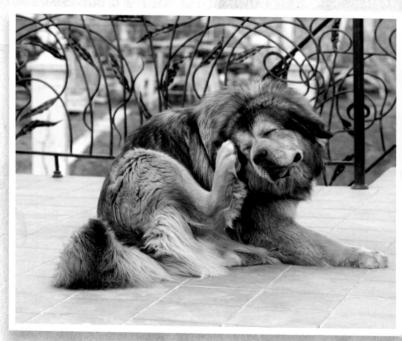

Use ACV for itchy skin

ITCHY SKIN

For any patches of itchy skin on your dog, mix a solution of 1 part ACV and 1 part water in a spray bottle and apply directly onto itchy patches. If you can't apply the mixture topically and the itchy skin is result of yeast, add ¼ to ½ teaspoon ACV to your dog's food or water twice daily.

WARNING!
Do NOT apply ACV to open wounds.

For a more general fix, try combining 3 tablespoons ACV with 1 quart water to make a soothing post-bath rinse. After bathing your dog as usual, pour the ACV mixture over your dog's coat. Be sure to avoid getting the mixture into your dog's eyes! There is no need to rinse; simply towel-dry your dog and then let air dry.

Tip: ACV should never be consumed undiluted; this is doubly true for your pets.

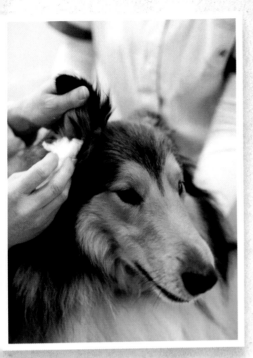

Remove wax buildup

CLEAN EARS

Make a mixture of 1 part ACV and 1 part water to make a natural ear cleaning solution. Simply soak a cotton ball in your ACV mixture and use it to clean out wax buildup in your dog's ear. The antibacterial properties of ACV can help to treat yeast-based ear infections; make sure that the inside of the ear is not raw prior to using ACV to treat an ear infection.

REPEL FLEAS AND TICKS

Spray your dog with a mixture of 1 part ACV and 1 part water to help repel ticks and fleas. Be sure to continue to do flea and tick checks after your dog has been playing outside!

WARNING!

When swabbing your dog's ear, only go in as far as you can see to avoid damage.

SOOTHE SORE PAWS

In a large bowl, combine 1 part ACV with 2 parts water. Soak your dog's paws for up to 5 minutes and thoroughly dry them with a towel; there is no need to rinse.

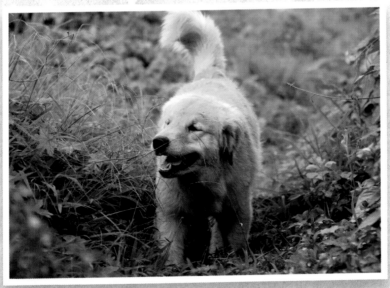

Soak your dog's paws

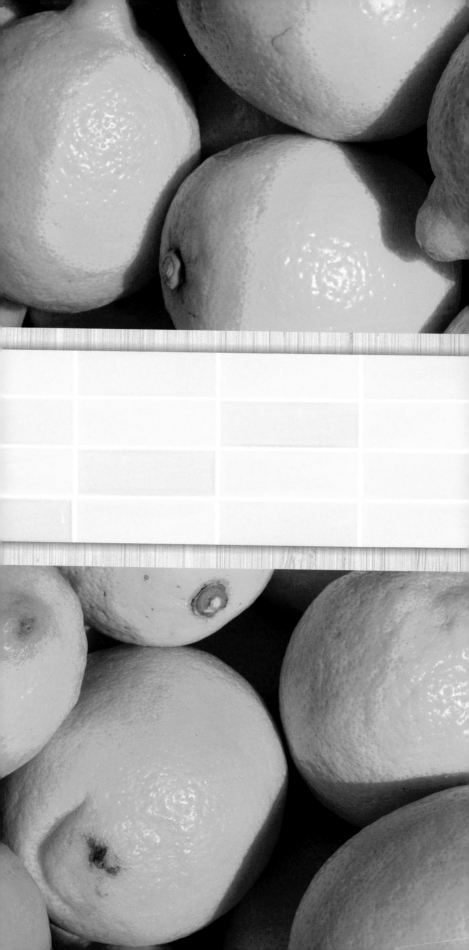

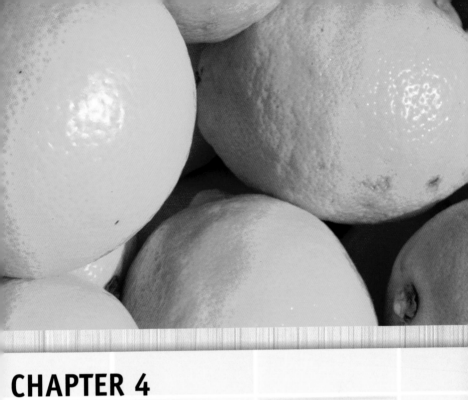

CHAPTER 4
LEMONS

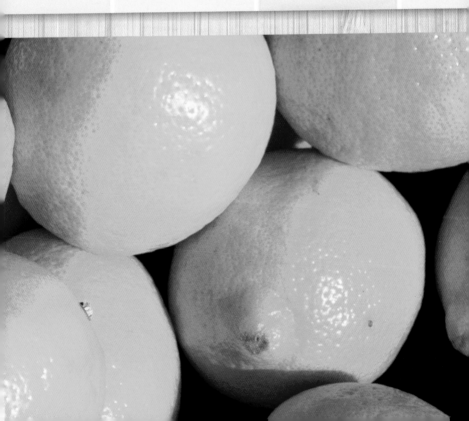

LEMON USES

Lemons are one of nature's most versatile fruits, with uses ranging from preserving food to acting as a natural weed killer. Because of the acidic nature of lemons, they can be used to clean, deodorize, or disinfect just about anything. You can bleach your hair, clean your oven, fight a cold, and exfoliate your skin, all with this one ingredient. If you want to avoid toxic cleaning products, expensive skin and hair-care regimens, and keep yourself feeling fit and healthy, pick up a few lemons next time you go grocery shopping and put them to work.

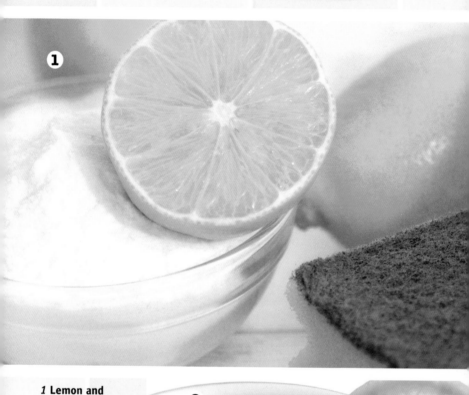

1 **Lemon and baking soda**
2 **Lemon tea**
3 **Lemons and salt**
4 **Lemon juice**
5 **Lemon face rinse**
6 **Fresh lemon**

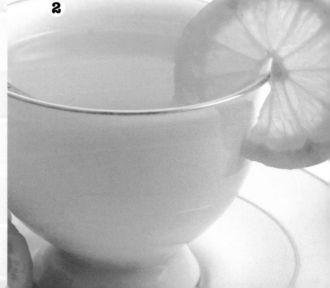

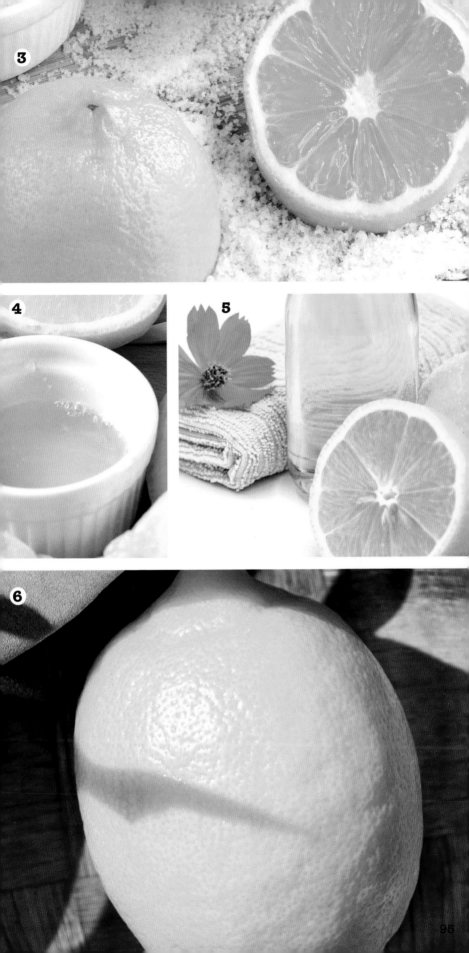

WELLNESS

You need to maintain a good balance of fruits and vegetables in your diet to stay healthy and energized, and citrus fruits like oranges, grapefruit, and lemons have some very well-known health benefits. Lemons in particular, however, have a number of other uses that help promote physical and mental well-being that not many people know about.

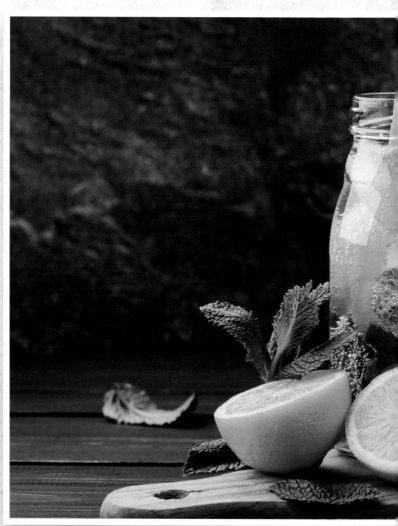

Lemons can be a powerful dietary supplement

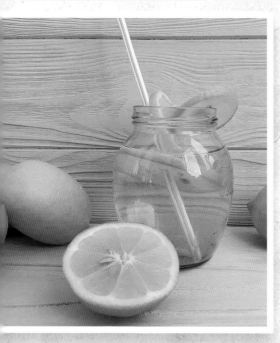

From boosting your immune system to fighting dandruff to helping treat poison ivy—as well as simply carrying a surprising amount of nutritional benefits—you'll soon find that lemons are a helpful fruit indeed.

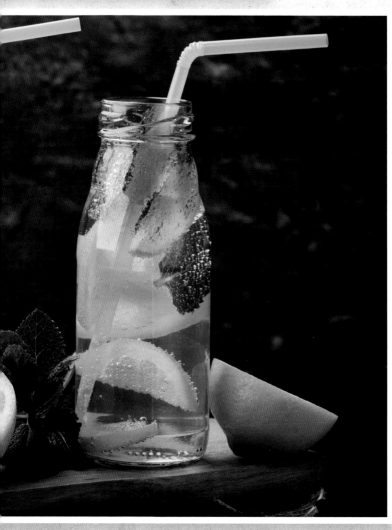

WELLNESS

The best way to get a whole cadre of health benefits from lemons all at once is to drink lemon water or lemon tea several times a day. You might want to start the day by squeezing half a lemon into a glass of warm water, or making a cup of tea with honey and lemon to kick off the day. You can also drink lemon water before each meal, to help with digestion and to keep your metabolism going strong.

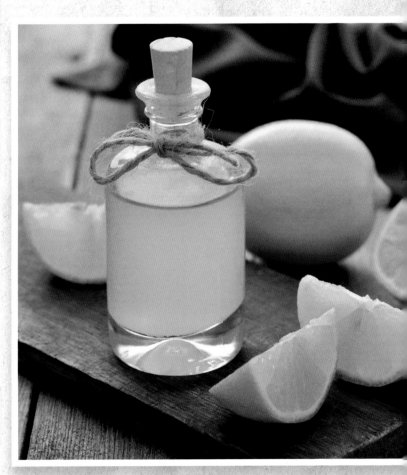

Raw lemon juice

AVOID KIDNEY STONES

One of the great benefits of adding a glass or two of lemon water to your daily routing is that the acidity of lemon juice helps your body avoid the formation of kidney stones. Citrate, a compound that helps break down kidney stones and keep them from forming in the first place, is present in high quantities in lemons and lemon juice, allowing a regular intake of lemon water to serve as both a preventative and curative measure.

IMMUNE SYSTEM

Lemons are a good source of vitamin C, which is necessary to keep your body's immune system up and running. If you regularly drink lemon water or lemon tea, that's one less dietary requirement to worry about, and you'll be less likely to get sick with a stronger immune system.

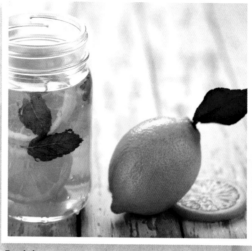

Fresh lemon water

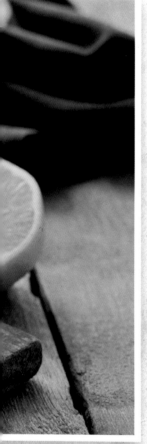

ENERGY BOOSTER

You can use a glass of lemon water as a natural, healthy alternative to your morning energy drink or cup of coffee. Lemon juice is high in electrolytes, which are instrumental in revitalizing you when you're low on energy. The smell and taste of lemons are also associated with increased moods and feelings of energy, which can also help give you a boost in the morning.

AID DIGESTION

Another reason to drink lemon water every morning and before each meal is to help kick-start your metabolism, aiding in digestion throughout the rest of your day. Drinking a glass of water—especially room temperature or warm water, to help your body absorb it more quickly—every morning will always help your digestive system get started faster and work more efficiently, and adding fresh-squeezed lemon juice to that water will help stimulate the production of stomach acid. Lemon juice is also a diuretic, which will promote further hydration and help flush out

LOWER BLOOD PRESSURE

Hypertension, or high blood pressure, can be controlled in part by a regular intake of lemons and/or lemon juice. Lemons are high in vitamin C, help act as an antioxidant, and reduce cholesterol—all of which can contribute to lowering blood pressure and improving heart health.

WELLNESS

TREAT SORE THROATS

One of the oldest, most tried and true methods of treating sore throats, colds, and coughs is a hot mug of lemon tea with honey. Juice a whole lemon or two, depending on how strong you want your tea to be, and mix it into a mug of boiling water along with a few teaspoons of honey.

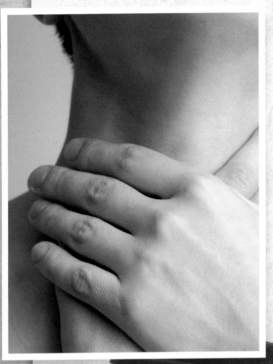

The honey helps soothe the pain of a sore throat, especially if it's been further irritated by long bouts of coughing, and the acid of the lemon juice helps break up mucus and kill some of the bacteria that is most likely causing your sore throats and colds in the first place. Drinking more water is also always a good way to help recover from a cold, so this should be a multi-faceted way to help bring yourself back up to speed.

Soothe a sore throat

TREAT HEADACHES

If you regularly suffer from headaches or migraines, you might want to try this mixture of lemon juice, water, and salt to help alleviate the pain. Mix 2 teaspoons salt, one thoroughly juiced lemon, and 1 cup warm water together and drink while still warm (but not hot). This drink should help improve your electrolyte balance and rehydrate you, alleviating one of the most common causes of headaches. If you use high quality salt, such as Himalayan sea salt, the magnesium content present should also act as a minor pain reliever.

DISINFECT CUTS AND SCRAPES

While it might sting quite a bit, you can use lemon juice to help disinfect small cuts, scrapes, and burns. Lemon is a natural antiseptic given its acidic properties, which helps fight bacteria and keep cuts from getting infected. It may also help slow the bleeding of small wounds.

WARNING!

It's generally advisable to use medical-grade antiseptic on cuts and scrapes if you have it available. You should always consult a medical professional if you sustain an injury or acquire an illness greater than a small cut or a common cold.

TREAT POISON IVY

Undiluted lemon juice can also be used to help minimize the symptoms of an allergic reaction to poison ivy. Coating the affected area with lemon juice and then rinsing with cool or lukewarm water should help soothe the painful rash that comes with contact with poison ivy. If you can apply it soon enough after first touching the plant, the lemon juice may flush away some of the toxic oil, reducing the amount that reacts with your skin in the first place.

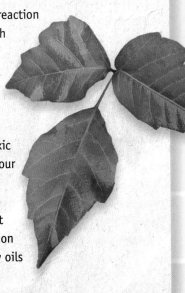

Generally, the pus from a poison ivy rash isn't infectious—only the oil from the plant itself. The only risk of spreading the infection comes from not thoroughly washing off any oils from the plant.

BEAUTY/PERSONAL

Lemon juice contains a number of useful components that make it great for your skin, hair, and more. While it is acidic, which allows it to help exfoliate and tone your skin and return a youthful glow to your appearance, the acidity of lemon juice is low enough to use pretty liberally without risk of damaging your skin. A skin care regimen that includes lemon juice—or even just lemon rinds, if you have especially sensitive skin—should leave your skin looking and feeling smoother, brighter, and cleaner. You can also make your own DIY facial scrubs, sun-bleach your hair for natural highlights, and even lose a little weight, all with little more than a few lemons.

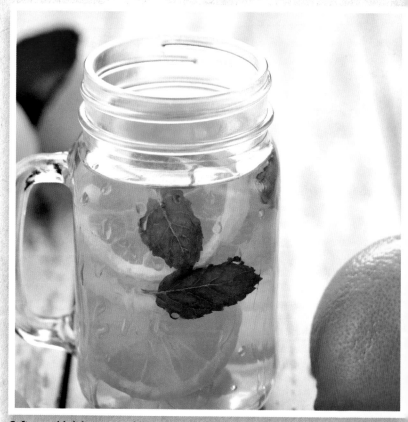

Soften and brighten your skin

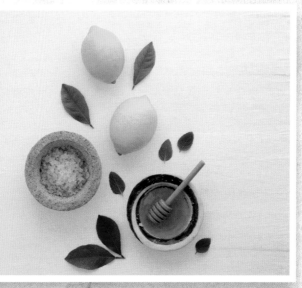

lemon, honey, and salt

NATURALLY BLEACH HAIR

One interesting way to use lemon juice cosmetically is to naturally sun-bleach your hair. All you have to do is comb or spray some lemon juice through clean, dry hair before leaving the house and spending a day in the sun. This should work best on bright, sunny summer days, and it's a great way to add some natural highlights to your hair.

Tip: Try mixing a little coconut oil with the lemon juice, to keep your hair from getting too dry.

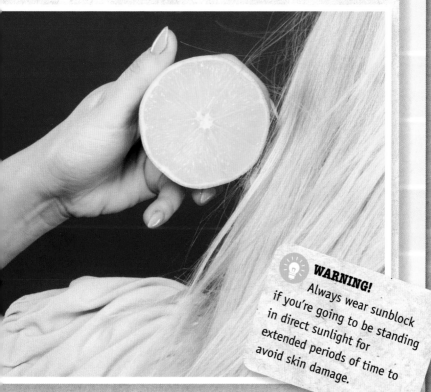

WARNING!
Always wear sunblock if you're going to be standing in direct sunlight for extended periods of time to avoid skin damage.

naturally bleach your hair

BEAUTY/PERSONAL

DANDRUFF

Lemon juice is a useful and cheap way to help fight dandruff, without having to spend the money on man-made solutions that might do more harm to your scalp and hair than good. Gently rub 2 tablespoons lemon juice into your scalp and roots, and rinse with warm water. You can also dilute the lemon juice in water if you have especially sensitive skin or delicate hair. The acidity of the lemon will help cut through an overabundance of oil in your scalp while also helping get rid of dead or dry skin. Continue this every day, and you should see results in no time.

Tip: Add 1 tablespoon coconut oil, tea tree oil, or apple cider vinegar to make your own personalized, more powerful dandruff treatment.

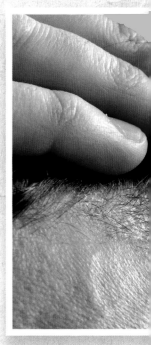

Fight dandruff

FACIAL SCRUB

You can make any number of face and body scrubs with lemon juice to exfoliate and tone your skin, reducing wrinkles and making your skin softer and smoother than ever. The simplest option is to simply mix together ½ a juiced lemon with ¼ cup sugar. You can make this scrub

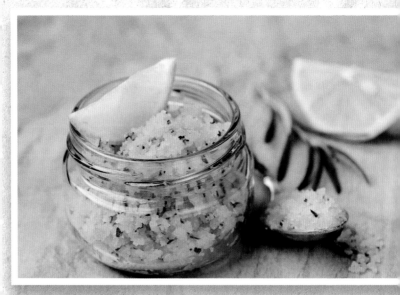

Lemon and sugar facial scrub

on a budget, and it will taste pretty good if you use it as a lip exfoliant, too. If you want to make your scrub a little more interesting, you can include just about anything you want, from honey to apple cider vinegar to coconut oil. A few drops of an essential oil of your choice might be a good addition, too.

BODY WAX

If you need an alternative body wax that isn't quite as painful as traditional waxing, you can use lemons to make a sugar wax that should remove hair at the root without irritating the skin underneath. On the stove, mix together 1 cup sugar, ¼ cup lemon juice, and ¼ cup water. Heat the mixture on medium, stirring continuously, until it's reached a golden-brown, honey-like consistency. Pour the wax into a bowl or jar, and allow it to cool for 30 minutes. Then, simply use your sugar wax the same way you would normally wax, without the risk of bleeding or skin damage.

Tip: Sugar wax is just as malleable and sticky when cool, so you should make sure to let it cool down before use to avoid burning yourself.

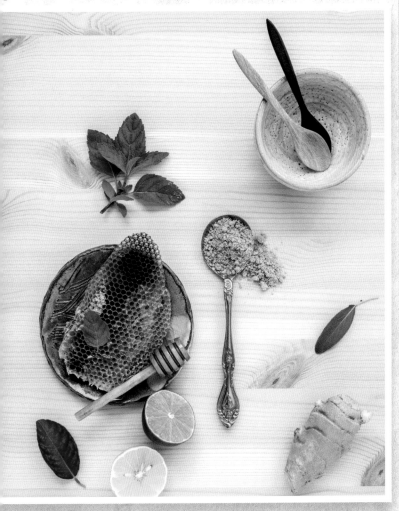

emon and beeswax

BEAUTY/PERSONAL

NAILS

You can use lemon juice as a way to return dull fingernails to a glossy shine in just a few minutes without a costly manicure. The easiest way is to soak your fingernails for up to five minutes at a time in a bowl of lemon juice, or to buff your fingernails with a cut lemon for several minutes at a time. You can also mix together lemon juice with either salt or sugar, making an exfoliating scrub to shine your nails and remove dead skin around your cuticles.

Tip: Moisturize your hands and fingernails after using lemon to keep them in good shape.

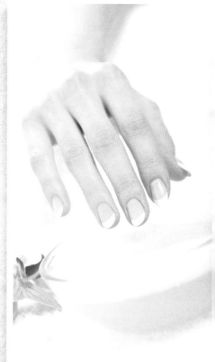

Shine your nails

TEETH

If your teeth are discolored by smoking, drinking coffee, or poor dental hygiene, there are a few quick, effective ways to whiten your teeth with lemon juice. First, you might want to try brushing your teeth with diluted lemon juice: combine in a glass 1 teaspoon water for every teaspoon of lemon juice, dip your toothbrush in, and brush your teeth vigorously for a minute or so. Make sure to rise thoroughly and follow up with regular toothpaste. You can also use a lemon peel instead—rub the inside of a lemon peel against your teeth

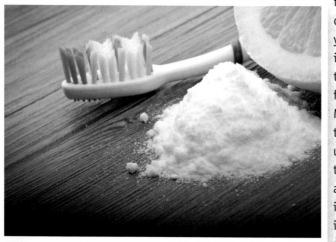

Whiten teeth

for several minutes as though brushing your teeth, and then rinse with water as before.

EYE BAGS

You can use a mixture of lemon and cucumber juice to rejuvenate the skin under your eyes and minimize the shadows and bruising that occur when you don't get enough sleep. Simply combine 1 teaspoon lemon juice and 1 teaspoon cucumber juice in a small jar and gently apply it to your cheeks and lower eyelids. Leave on for 5–15 minutes before washing your face clean.

Tip: Try mixing in some coconut oil to help rehydrate and rejuvenate your skin a little more.

WARNING!

If you have sensitive teeth, using acidic substances like lemon juice can wear away the enamel on your teeth. A more diluted solution combined with regular use of enamel-protecting toothpaste should help keep your teeth healthy. Always consult a dentist or doctor first if you have any health concerns.

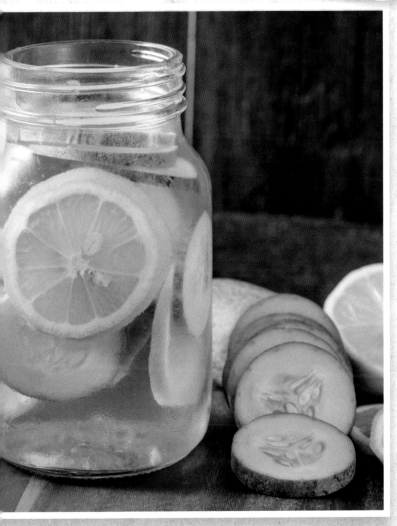

Reduce eye bags

BEAUTY/PERSONAL

SKIN HEALTH
Age spots

Age spots can be unsightly and annoying, but products that are on the market that claim to remove them can be full of harmful chemicals, as well as being pretty expensive. Lemon juice is a cheaper, natural way to help lighten dark spots and discoloration caused by aging. The acid in lemons helps lighten spots and exfoliates skin, which can help reduce and prevent signs of aging.

To try this method for yourself, soak a cotton ball in fresh lemon juice and dab on dark spots once to twice daily. Allow the juice to remain on skin for at least 30 minutes.

WARNING!

Avoid going out the sun with lemon jui your skin. Sunlight can the lemon juice irritate a possibly damage your skin Wait a few minutes after applying the lemon juice before exposing your skin to sunlight.

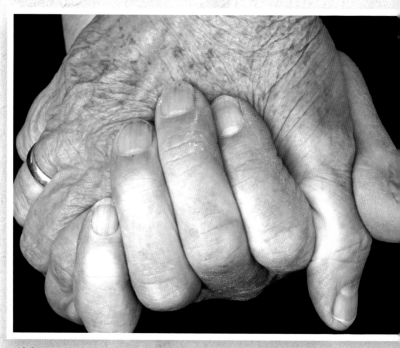

Lighten age spots with lemon

Acne

If you struggle with acne, lemon juice might be exactly what you need to get your skin feeling healthy and smooth again. Start by washing your face with gentle soap and warm water, and dry with a soft towel or washcloth. Then, all you have to do is use a cotton ball, washcloth, or clean paper towel to apply fresh-squeezed lemon juice to any affected areas.

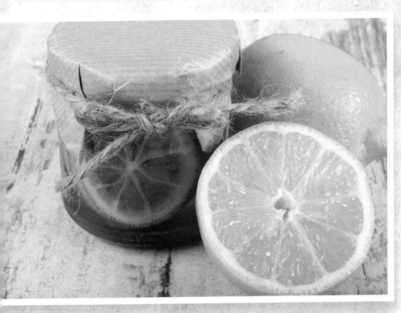

raw lemon juice

FRESHEN BREATH

Bad breath is one of the first things a person will notice when you're having a conversation with them, so it is important to fix it as soon as possible. Many natural toothpastes that are sold are great for protecting your teeth, however they are not very effective at fighting bad breath. Luckily, lemon juice is a natural, time proven remedy that will freshen your breath in no time. Simply mix 1 tablespoon lemon juice into a cup of lukewarm water with a pinch of salt. Stir this and use it to rinse your mouth. The acid from the lemon juice will kill any bacteria in your mouth that causes bad breath, and the salt will prevent your mouth from getting dry.

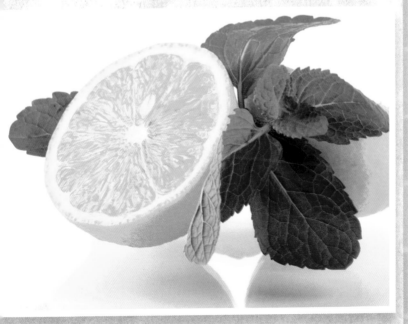

freshen breath

BEAUTY/PERSONAL

SOFTEN HANDS AND FEET

Rough hands and feet can be annoying and embarrassing, and skin cracking caused by roughness can lead to cuts that can risk infection. This makes it very important to combat roughness on hands and feet, but sometimes even the strongest lotions and creams are not effective. The good news is that there is an easy way to soften your hands and feet, by making a natural scrub using lemon juice and sugar. All you need to do is mix 1 tablespoon lemon juice, ½ cup brown sugar, 1 teaspoon honey, and ½ cup olive oil. Soak your hands and feet in warm water for about 20 minutes, then gently scrub with the mixture you made. Rinse off with warm water and pat dry.

Tip: Once your skin is soft and smooth again, apply moisturizer generously to hands and feet, then put on socks and gloves over the moisturizer so that it can absorb into your skin better.

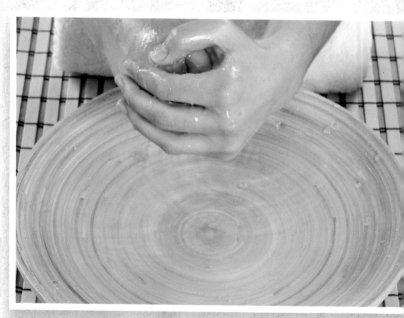

Soften skin with lemons

LOSE WATER WEIGHT

For many people struggling with their weight, the first problem they need to overcome is water retention. Your body will retain water for a lot of reasons, including stress, too much salt consumption, and not enough water consumption. Water retention can cause you to gain weight, even if you're exercising and trying to eat healthily. Lemons can help with this problem in a couple different ways. Adding lemons to your water and drinking it at the beginning of the day and throughout the day can stop your body from retaining water. This works because

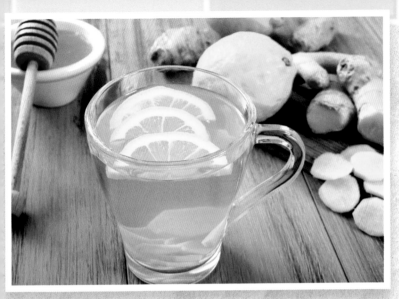

Lemon and honey tea

your body will be getting more water every day, and the lemon helps act as a diuretic to remove the excess water from your body. Adding lemons to water also helps trick you into drinking more water, because it will taste better than plain water alone. It also will help you cut out sugary drinks, since the lemon will provide you with the sweet taste you crave.

REMOVE WARTS

The standard procedure to remove warts can be pretty painful. While nothing will be as quick as chemically freezing off the wart, lemon juice is a gentler option for do-it-yourself removal. The acid from the lemons will gradually break down the wart, and with daily applications, the wart will go away in a couple of weeks. Soak a cotton ball in fresh lemon juice, then let it sit on top of the wart. Dab at the wart a few times, but do not rinse the lemon juice off. Do this twice a day until the wart disappears.

Tip: To increase the effectiveness of the lemon juice method, try applying very finely chopped onions to the wart for about 15 minutes.

PSORIASIS

Psoriasis can cause itchy, painful, and embarrassing flare-ups for people who are diagnosed with this autoimmune disorder. Many sufferers spend hours a day applying ointment to their rashes and taking medication, only for the symptoms to never fully go away. Some people have bad reactions to the medications prescribed, but continue to suffer, thinking that they have no other options. Some psoriasis sufferers, however, have found that lemons can provide a surprising amount of relief from their symptoms. Because lemons help to protect and strengthen the immune system, they are very useful to those with immune system problems. Adding lemons to water and teas can help prevent flare-ups, and applying lemon juice directly to rashes can help them go away more quickly and not progress into a more painful lesion.

HOME

Once you've gotten into the habit of using lemons to maintain your personal health and appearance, you can also use them to clean up the space around you. Lemon juice can be used to clean and disinfect just about anything you can think of, deodorize musty carpets and stained clothes, and even scour away rust, all while allowing you to avoid harsher and more expensive artificial cleaners. When you clean with lemon juice, you also get the benefit of filling your house with the fresh scent of citrus, making everything smell cleaner and giving your mood a boost.

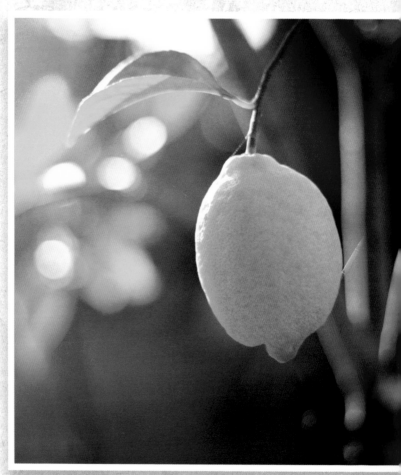

Lemon juice helps kill bacteria and fight stains

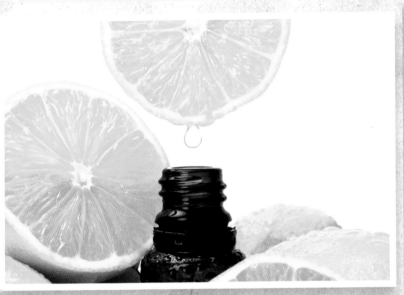

Lemon juice

MAKE AN ALL-PURPOSE CLEANER

The acidity of lemons makes them a great option for all kinds of cleaning. While different jobs might need slightly different concentrations or ingredients, you can make a powerful all-purpose cleaner for daily use with just lemons, white vinegar, and water.

In a glass jar or a clear plastic spray bottle, mix 2 cups white vinegar, 2 cups water, and the juice and rinds of ½ lemon. Leave the mixture to sit for about 2 weeks in a cool spot out of direct sunlight, and then transfer to a spray bottle.

Tip: For best results, wait for a few seconds after spraying your cleaner onto a surface before wiping it away, to give it time to work.

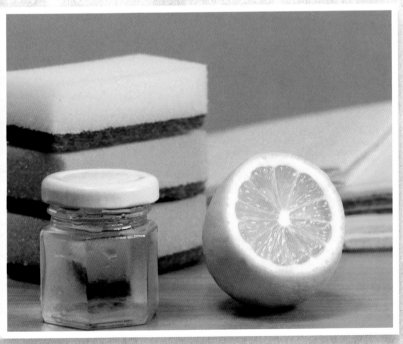

Lemon all-purpose cleaner

HOME

CLEAN AND DEODORIZE GARBAGE DISPOSALS

Garbage disposals are convenient and useful parts of our kitchen, but it is in their nature to attract odors and bacteria. Unfortunately, cleaning them is not as easy as the other surfaces in your kitchen, and trying to clean them can be dangerous. Fortunately, there is an easy, natural way to deodorize your garbage disposal and kill the bacteria that can live in it. Deodorizing pods can be made by mixing ¾ cup baking soda, ½ cup table salt, ½ teaspoon dishwashing soap, and the zest of 1 lemon. Add about 3 tablespoons lemon juice until the mixture looks like slightly wet sand. Pack tightly into an empty ice cube tray and allow to dry overnight. Remove pods and store in an airtight container. When ready to use, drop one pod into the garbage disposal and turn on. Using these as needed will help keep your garbage disposal as clean and odor free as the rest of your kitchen.

GLASS CLEANER

From mirrors to windows to sliding doors, glass is everywhere in our houses, and if you have small children or pets, these glass objects can never seem to stay smudge free. Store-bought glass cleaners work well enough, but they are full of harsh chemicals and dyes that can be dangerous to your family, especially if you need to use them often. These chemicals can also damage other, non-glass surfaces in your house. However, there is a natural, effective alternative that you can make using lemon juice. Simply add 3 tablespoons lemon juice and ½

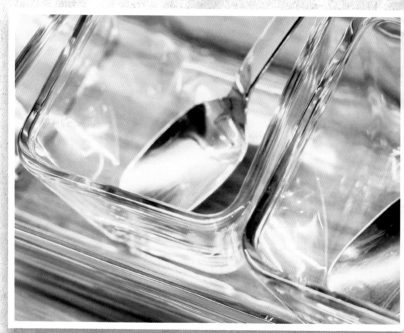

Clean glassware with lemons

cup rubbing alcohol to a spray bottle. Fill the bottle the rest of the way with water and shake well to mix.

CLEAN TOILETS

Toilet bowls are one of the dirtiest places in a home, and keeping them clean can be a real chore. Commercial toilet cleaners are also one of the most dangerous home cleaners, as they can cause burns if they get on your skin and the fumes can be harmful for you and your family. An easy and much less dangerous solution can be made using lemon juice and borax. All you need to do is sprinkle ¼ cup borax into the toilet bowl. Squeeze the juice of ½ lemon into the bowl. Let the mixture sit in the bowl for a few minutes. Scrub with a brush, then flush.

SCOUR RUST

As metal objects get older, they tend to rust. This is unsightly and unsafe, especially when the rust is on kitchen appliances. Rust is notoriously difficult to remove, and commercial rust cleaners are full of dangerous chemicals. Scraping the rust off can cause the rust to go into the air, which can be breathed in accidentally. Luckily, all you really need to remove it is a lemon and some coarse salt. Rub a liberal amount of salt over the rusted area. Squeeze or spray lemon juice over the whole area, and allow to sit for about 3 hours. Then, scrub the area with lemon rinds to remove the rust.

REMOVE SWEAT STAINS

White t-shirts are particularly prone to getting unpleasant yellow sweat stains that can seem impossible to remove. Often, commercial stain removers will not work for these types of stains, and using bleach can ruin other clothes in the wash. Lemon juice, however, can work as a bleaching agent without ruining your laundry. All you need to do is fill a spray bottle with pure, undiluted lemon juice. Before washing a shirt with sweat stains, spray the stains thoroughly with the lemon juice. Then, wash the shirt as you would normally, and the stains should fade.

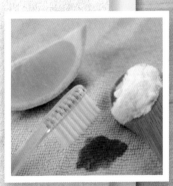

Create organic cleaners by mixing baking soda and lemon for stains

DEODORIZE CARPETS

Make your own carpet deodorizer by combining 2 cups baking soda with 20 drops lemon essential oil. Sprinkle the mixture over the whole carpet and allow to sit for about 15 minutes, longer for dirtier carpets. Then, simply vacuum up the powder and enjoy your fresh new carpet. Store in a shaker jar for easy use.

Tip: For an even fresher scent, add about 5 drops of another essential oil, such as thyme or rosemary, to the mixture.

HOME

WHITEN CLOTHES

Traditional methods of whitening clothes by using chlorine-based bleach can be dangerous and harmful to your health. Bleach fumes should not be breathed in, and if bleach gets on your skin it can cause painful irritation. It also smells terrible, and many bleach products have added fragrances to try to mask that smell, and these fragrances can stay in your clothes and cause irritation when you where them. Lemon juice, on the other hand, is a natural alternative to chlorine bleach that smells great and is far less dangerous. Simply add ¼ cup lemon juice to your load of whites during the rinse cycle. Dry the clothes in the sun to activate the brightening effects of the lemon juice.

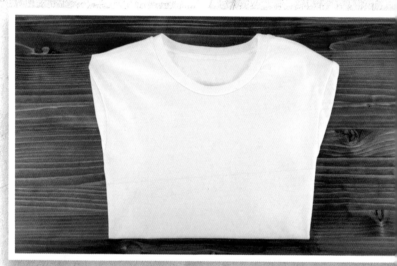

Remove stains

NEUTRALIZE ONION HANDS

Chopping onions won't just make you cry, it can also give your hands an unpleasant odor that can linger well after you've washed your hands. An easy way to remove these odors is by rubbing lemon rinds between your hands. The rinds act as a gentle scouring agent, which will remove onions' oils left on your hands. The lemon will also leave behind a pleasant scent.

CLEAN MICROWAVE

Place ½ lemon, cut side up, in a bowl. Fill bowl with water and place in the microwave. Microwave on high for 5 minutes. Grime and stains should easily wipe off the inside surface of the microwave. If it does not, microwave the bowl for another five minutes.

Tip: Add 20 drops of your favorite essential oil to the water before microwaving to deodorize the microwave.

PRESERVE BROWNING FRUITS

To preserve cut fruits and vegetables and prevent them from turning brown, put the cut pieces in a container and sprinkle with lemon juice. This will help them keep longer in the refrigerator than the cut produce would last alone.

Tip: When saving a halved piece of any fruit, you can put ½ lemon against the cut side of the fruit and use a rubber band to keep them together. This will prevent the fruit from browning, and you won't need a container to put it in.

Preserve fruits

REPEL INSECTS

The smell of lemons can help repel ants. The lemon scent covers the scent tracks they use to communicate where to go. There are three methods to use lemons to prevent ants from entering your home and pantries.

• Soak a washcloth in lemon juice and wipe down all areas where you think ants are entering the house.

• Leave lemon rinds around outside doorways to repel ants.

• Soak cotton balls with lemon essential oil and place in cabinets where food is kept.

KILL WEEDS

Douse pure lemon juice on weeds. After a day or two, the lemon juice paired with light from the sun will cause the weeds to shrivel and die.
Tip: For weeds that will not die, try mixing 1 part white vinegar per 1 part lemon juice and dousing the weeds again.

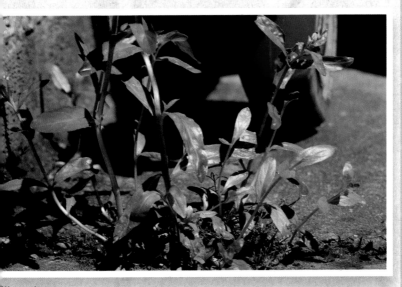

ll weeds

HOME

LAUNDRY DETERGENT

To make homemade, natural laundry detergent pods, you will need 1 bar castile soap, 1 cup washing soda, ¼ cup Epsom salt, ½ cup white vinegar, and 10–20 drops lemon essential oil. Grate the soap using a food processor or the fine side of a hand grater. Combine dry ingredients in a bowl, then add the lemon essential oil. Add the vinegar tablespoon by tablespoon until the mixture is clumpy and packable. Pack the mixture into an ice cube tray and allow to sit for at least 24 hours. Store in an airtight container and use one pod for a regular sized load of laundry.

Tip: If you don't have washing soda, you can make some by placing baking soda in a thin layer on a baking sheet, then baking at 400°F for about 40 minutes.

WASH FRUITS AND VEGETABLES

Fruits and vegetables that we buy from the grocery store are usually sprayed with pesticides and waxes to keep them fresh and looking nice. However, consuming these pesticides can make you and your family sick. To remove them before eating, simply mix 1 tablespoon

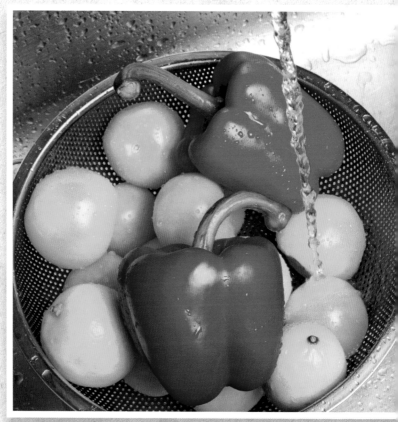

Keep produce clean

lemon juice with 2 tablespoons baking soda and 1 cup water. Whisk the mixture until the baking soda is completely dissolved. Pour the mixture into a spray bottle, then spray produce until it is completely soaked. Let the mixture sit on the produce for about 5 minutes, then rinse thoroughly and dry.

Tip: Use this spray on organic produce and produce that you grow yourself as well. While the organic produce may not be sprayed with pesticides, it could have topical bacteria which will be killed using this spray.

CLEAN HUMIDIFIERS

Even with regular cleaning, humidifiers can need a little extra treatment to prevent the growth of bacteria, mold, and mildew. A natural way to do this is by adding 1 tablespoon fresh lemon juice to the water in the humidifier every time you fill it. The lemon juice will kill bacteria that can grow in the water, and will release a pleasant scent into the air as well.

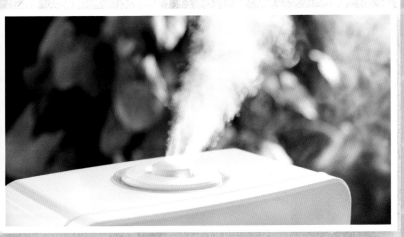

Clean humidifiers

CLEAN MILDEWED CLOTHES

Mildew can grow anywhere there is a damp place without ventilation, such as a child's sports locker. It can be smelly and annoying, and sometimes mildew can be a hazard to your health. It can seem to be impossible to remove from fabric, and you might be tempted to just throw the item away. However, there is a natural solution for removing mildew from clothes. Due to its antifungal properties, lemon juice works very well at removing mildew. Simply add salt to ⅓ cup fresh lemon juice to form a paste, then rub the paste into the fabric. If necessary, scrub the paste in using an old toothbrush. Then wash the fabric as normal.

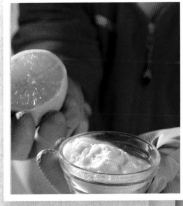

Remove mildew with lemons

HOME

STOP RICE CLUMPING

Rice is a favorite food staple for families all over the world, because it is tasty, inexpensive, and only a small amount is needed to make a large meal. However, rice can sometimes be a hassle to work with. Whether you cook your rice on the stovetop or in a special rice cooker, rice tends to be very sticky and clump together, which can make it difficult to work with. To loosen the rice grains and make it less sticky and clumpy, just add 1 tablespoon lemon juice to the water before cooking your rice and cook as normal. This will keep the rice fluffy and less sticky, and it will also help make the rice a brighter, more appetizing color.

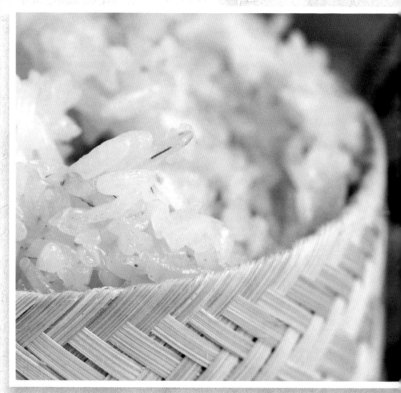

Stop rice from clumping

STOP BROWN SUGAR CLUMPING

Brown sugar is a necessity in any home where people love to bake, but the moisture in the sugar can cause it to become hard and difficult to scoop. Too many people end up throwing away their brown sugar because of clumping, which makes the sugar unusable. To prevent this

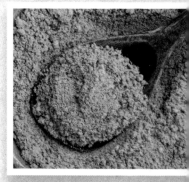

Brown sugar

waste, simply add dried lemon rinds from 1 lemon to your brown sugar container. This will prevent clumping and keep the sugar loose and easy to scoop.

KEEP LETTUCE CRISP

We all want to eat healthier, and fresh salads are a great way to do just that. However, many times lettuce starts to wilt

Crisp lettuce

before it can be eaten, causing much of it to go to waste. Even in the refrigerator, lettuce browns easily, making it unappetizing. An easy solution that will extend the life of your lettuce and keep it crisp and green uses lemon juice. All you need to do is soak the limp lettuce leaves in cold water with ½ cup lemon juice, then refrigerate for 1 hour. This will make the lettuce crisp again and ready to be made into a delicious salad.

KEEP GUACAMOLE GREEN AND FRESH

Leftover guacamole browns quickly, even when it's put in an airtight container in the refrigerator. To prevent this from happening, sprinkle lemon juice over the top of the guacamole, then cover and put in the

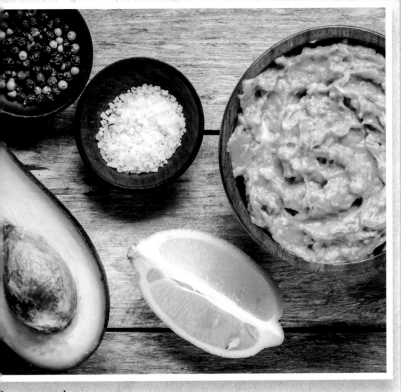

Keep guacamole green

HOME

fridge. The lemon juice stops the avocado from oxidizing, which is what causes it to brown, and you also get the added benefit of adding an interesting, citrusy kick to your dish.

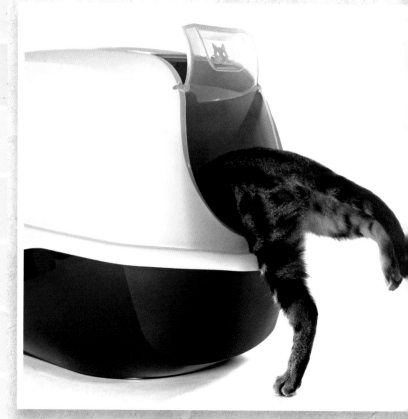

Freshen a litter box

DEODORIZE CAT LITTER BOX

To minimize the odor of a litter box that's staring to smell, mix 1 cup baking soda and about 20 drops lemon essential oil in a jar with a lid. Close the jar and shake to combine. Sprinkle the mixture in the litter box when you add more litter or whenever you clean it out.

POLISH METAL

Lemons make a great, cheap way to polish metal without having to use harsh or expensive chemical solutions. All you need is 1 lemon, some coarse sea salt, and a soft cloth. Cut your lemon in half, and coat the cut side of the lemon with an even layer of coarse sea salt. Use that side of the lemon to scrub whatever metal object you like until it shines as though brand new. Add more salt if the lemon juice starts to run out. When you're done, wipe the metal clean with a soft, slightly damp cloth and dry thoroughly.

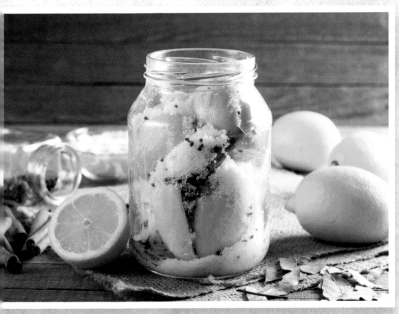

Lemons make a great, cheap way to polish metal without having to use harsh or expensive chemical solutions.

OVEN CLEANER

If you want to clean all the accumulated grime from an oven or stovetop, lemon juice is a good way to go. Mix 1 cup lemon juice with 2 cups white vinegar in a jar, bowl, or spray bottle, depending on how you intend to apply the mixture to your appliances. Spray or pour the lemon and vinegar onto any oven surfaces that need cleaning, let it sit for about 5 minutes, then sprinkle the surface liberally with baking soda. Leave it alone for 10 more minutes, then wipe up with a cloth. The mixture will allow even the toughest baked-in debris to wipe clean without having to scrub much at all.

Tip: For any leftover messes that will not wipe away easily, dip ½ a lemon in baking soda. Use this to scrub away tougher grime and stains.

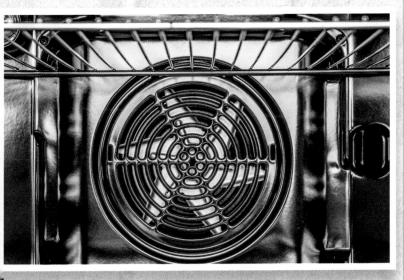

lean oven

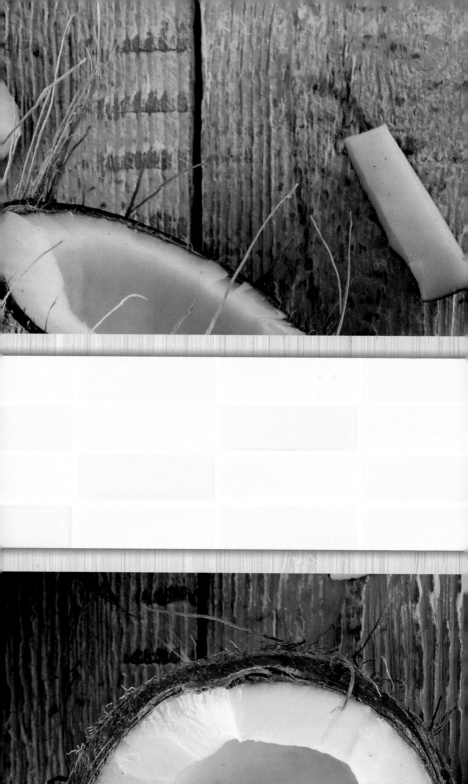
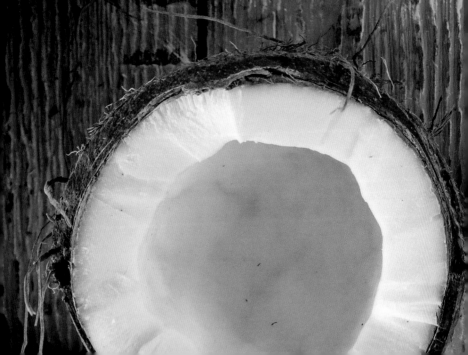

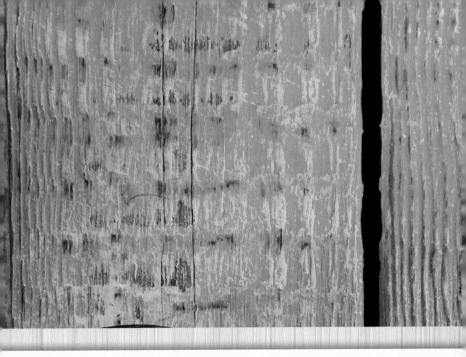

CHAPTER 5
COCONUT OIL

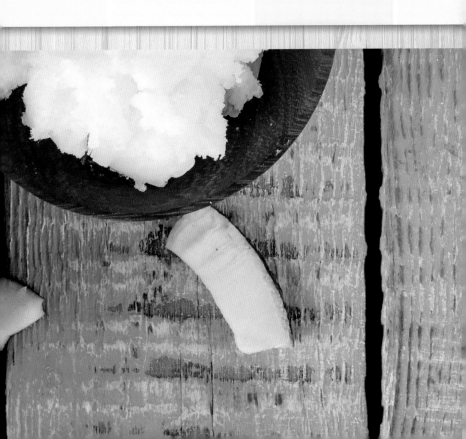

COCONUT OIL USES

Extracted from the meat of mature coconuts, coconut oil is an edible oil popular for cooking and baking. While coconut oil is tasty, its uses extend far beyond the kitchen. The antibacterial properties and unique fatty acid composition of coconut oil make it a versatile substance that can benefit your health and home.

Coconut milk is liquid that is harvested from the grated meat of a mature coconut. It is high in nutrients and has a wide range of health benefits. While coconut milk is best known for its benefits as a drink, it is also enormously beneficial for your skin and hair when applied topically.

Coconut water is a naturally occurring liquid that is found inside young coconuts. As the coconut matures, the water is replaced by coconut meat. Coconut water harvested from young coconuts contain the greatest nutrient health benefits.

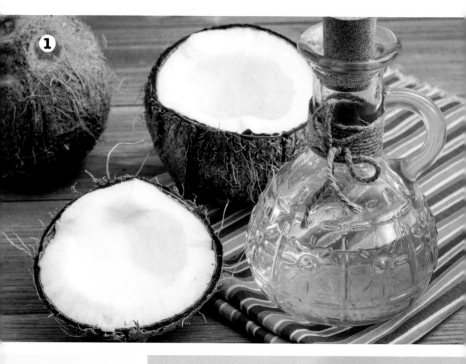

1 Coconuts
2 High in nutrients
3 Filtered coconut oil
4 Coconut water
5 Fresh coconut water
6 Raw coconut oil

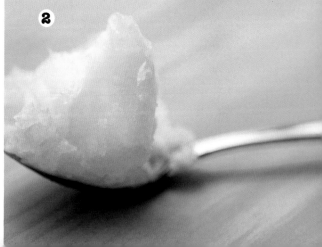

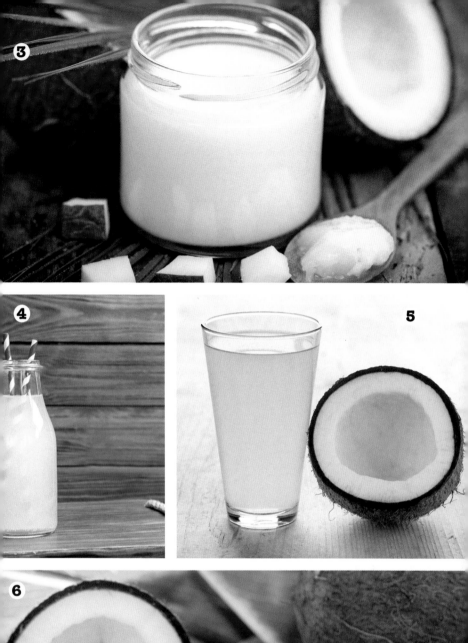
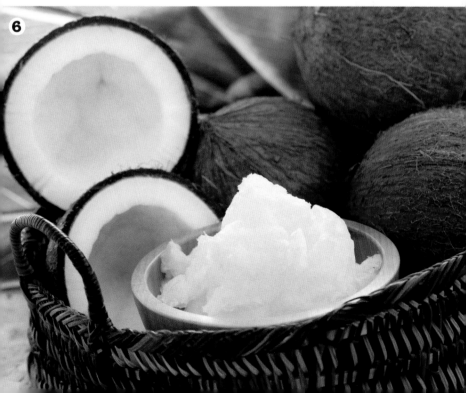

WELLNESS

Coconut oil is antibacterial and antifungal, making it a useful addition to your kitchen cabinet. Additionally, its unique composition of fatty acids can positively affect your health. Coconut oil is very moisturizing which, when combined with its antibacterial properties, makes it a good option to treat a variety of skin complaints.

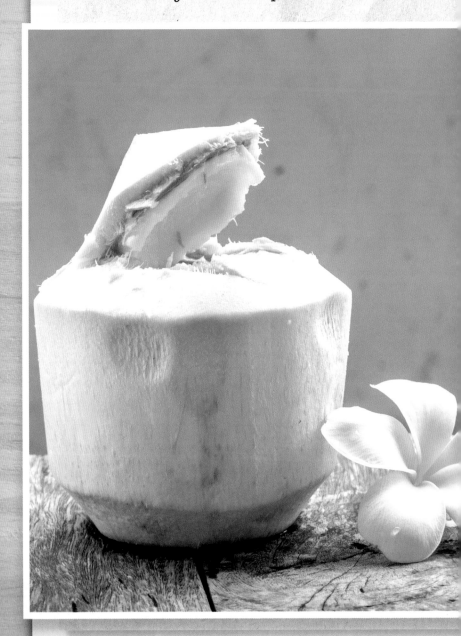

In many countries around the world, coconut oil has been used to maintain good oral hygiene and to keep hair and skin healthy. This versatile oil will become your new go-to for natural remedies.

COMBAT DIAPER RASH

The moisturizing, anti-inflammatory, and antibacterial properties of coconut oil make it a natural and efficient means of curing diaper rash in babies. Coconut oil can soothe the pain of diaper rash while simultaneously preventing further instances of the condition. You can use coconut oil alone by thoroughly washing and drying your baby's bottom and applying 1 teaspoon coconut oil directly to the affected area. You can also make your own coconut oil diaper cream.

Diaper Cream

½ cup organic, virgin coconut oil

¼ cup shea butter

1 teaspoon cornstarch

3–4 drops tea tree oil (optional)

Tip: Tree oil is great for treating yeast infections

In a small pot, combine coconut oil and shea butter and heat over a low flame until the mixture is liquified. Maintain the heat and slowly mix in the cornstarch while stirring. Once the cornstarch is mixed thoroughly, add the essential oil and stir. Store the finished product in a lidded glass jar or bottle.

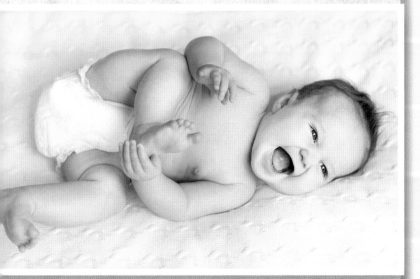

Ease diaper rash

Whether you use plain coconut oil or make your own diaper rash cream, be sure to apply the oil liberally onto clean, dry skin every time you change your baby's diaper.

WELLNESS

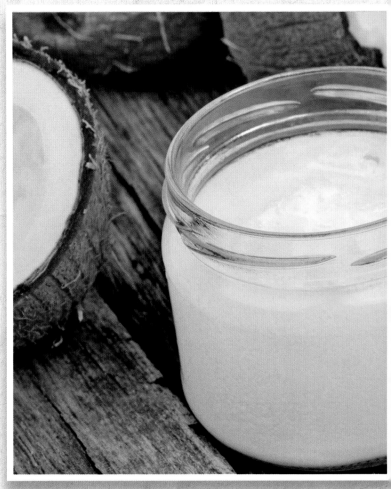

Coconut oil can be used as a natural moisurizer

FACE AND BODY MOISTURIZER

You can use coconut oil on your face and body as a natural moisturizer.
Coconut oil absorbs well, so you won't be left with greasy-feeling skin.
It can also boost collagen production, strengthening your skin.

Tip: Warm the coconut oil in your hands before applying to your face.
This will reduce the chance of clogging pores.

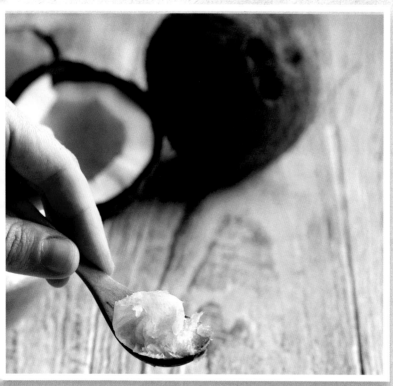

Fight bacteria

SUPPORT DIGESTION

The fats in coconut oil have well-known antimicrobial properties. By consuming 1 teaspoon coconut oil, you can combat indigestion as the oil's antimicrobial properties can help ward off bad bacteria, fungi, and parasites that hurt your stomach. Additionally, consuming coconut oil can aid your body in absorbing important vitamins, minerals, and amino acids

COMBAT A COLD

If you have a cold, you can make your own chest rub to combat congestion, headaches, and stuffy noses. Combine 2 tablespoons coconut oil, 5 drops eucalyptus oil, and 3 drops peppermint oil in a small bowl and stir. Apply the mixture to your chest with your fingers for quick symptom relief.

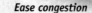

Ease congestion

131

WELLNESS

OIL PULLING

Oil pulling is an ancient Ayurvedic oral hygiene technique whereby you put 1 tablespoon coconut oil in your mouth and swish it around for 20 minutes. The idea behind this is that coconut oil can draw toxins from your body and salivary glands, improving oral health. When you spit the coconut oil out, you are also expelling the toxins.

The antibacterial and antifungal properties of coconut oil have been proven to be beneficial for oral hygiene, making it a natural, effective mouthwash.

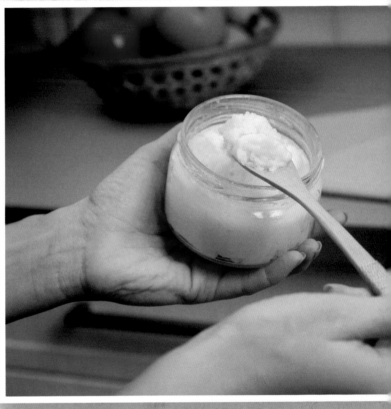

Coconut oil improves hygie

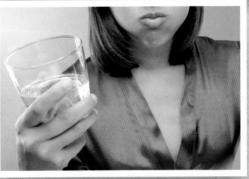

Swill coconut oil in your mouth

Tip: Spit the coconut oil into the trash, as it can clog your skink drain over time.

FIGHT INFLAMMATION

Studies have shown that coconut oil has anti-inflammatory and analgesic properties; its high levels of lauric acid mean that coconut oil can help reduce inflammation and potentially reduce pain levels. Additionally, topical application of coconut oil can increase blood supply to the area and reduce localized pain and swelling as a result of arthritis or other joint-pain conditions.

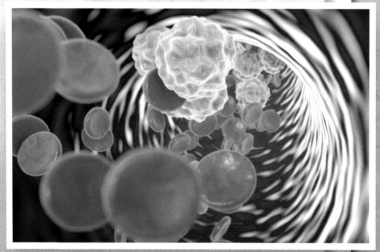

Overly abundant white blood cells, a cause of arthritis

BOOST IMMUNITY

Coconut oil contains high levels of lauric acid and caprylic acid, both of which are natural antibacterial, antiviral, and antifungal agents. These two acids are known to fight candida yeast overgrowth as well as some bacterial infections. Taking 1 teaspoon coconut oil orally once a day can boost your immunity. Try stirring it into your morning coffee, adding it to oatmeal or smoothies, or just taking it on its own.

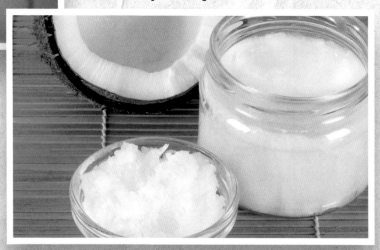

Coconut oil boosts immunity

WELLNESS

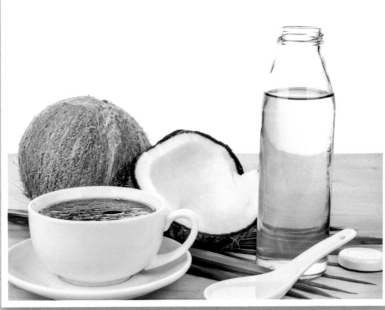

For most people, however, straight up eating a spoonful of fat seems excessive and is literally hard to swallow. Mixing coconut oil with your coffee, however, will make it go down like a treat.

SLEEP AID

While there are many reasons behind chronic insomnia or restless sleep in general, many times your disturbed sleep is caused by a spike in blood sugar that your liver doesn't have enough energy, or glycogen, to regulate your blood sugar levels throughout the night. When this happens, your adrenal glands produce adrenaline and cortisol which are stress hormones that can cause insomnia and poor quality sleep. Coconut oil contains

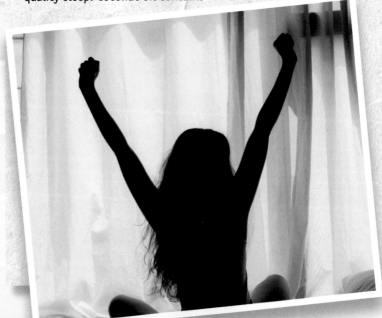

healthy fats that aide your body in producing sleep hormones like serotonin and melatonin, as well as helping you feel fuller longer so you don't wake up hungry.

When combined with raw honey, you can create a natural sleep aid to help you get to sleep faster and stay asleep longer. Raw honey produces glycogen, ensuring adequate liver glycogen stores, as well as stabilizes blood sugar levels, and contributes to the release of melatonin. Melatonin, while being a sleep hormone, also suppresses further blood sugar spikes, increasing the chance of an uninterrupted night's sleep.

Coconut and Honey Sleep Aid

1 tablespoon unrefined virgin coconut oil
½ teaspoon organic raw unfiltered honey

Combine the coconut oil and honey in a small bowl and mix. They can be difficult to combine, so be sure to stir thoroughly. Take 1 teaspoon of the mixture before bed. Store any excess in a small jar and keep by your bed; if you wake up in the night, you can take another spoonful to get back to sleep easier.

If you don't want to eat the mixture alone, try heating a small glass of milk (cow's milk, almond, cashew, coconut, etc.) and stirring in 1 teaspoon of the mixture. Drink before bedtime.

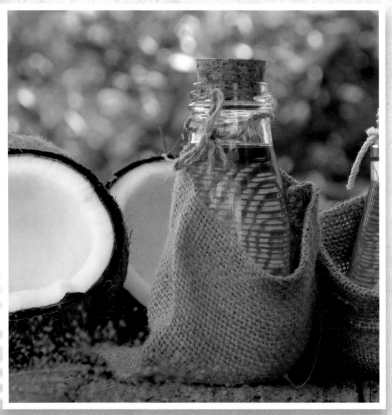

Harvested coconut oil

WELLNESS

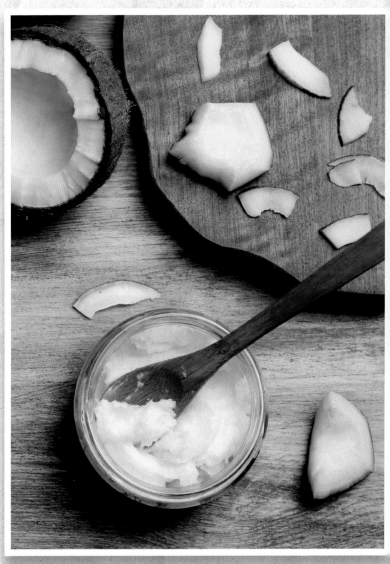

Consume coconut oil to burn fat

BURN FAT

Coconut oil contains a combination of medium-chain fatty acids, which are metabolized differently than longer chain fats, which is the type of fat found in most foods. Studies have shown that by adding coconut oil to your diet, you can lose fat. This is because medium-chain triglycerides—the fatty acids in coconut oil—are processed by the body differently and can boost metabolism. Try stirring 1 teaspoon coconut oil into your coffee in the morning. Additionally, coconut oil has a higher smoke point than olive oil or butter, making it a good choice for mid-temperature cooking.

ECZEMA AND PSORIASIS HELP

Coconut oil has antibacterial, antifungal, and antimicrobial properties that can help soothe your skin during an eczema or psoriasis flare-up, as well as reduce any inflammation. Additionally, the acids in coconut oil can fight against bacteria, fungi, and viruses, as well as help repair broken skin and keep your skin moisturized.

Apply a thin layer of organic extra virgin coconut oil directly to the affected area up to two times a day to help soothe flair ups, reduce the visibility of scarring, and help loosen psoriasis scales.

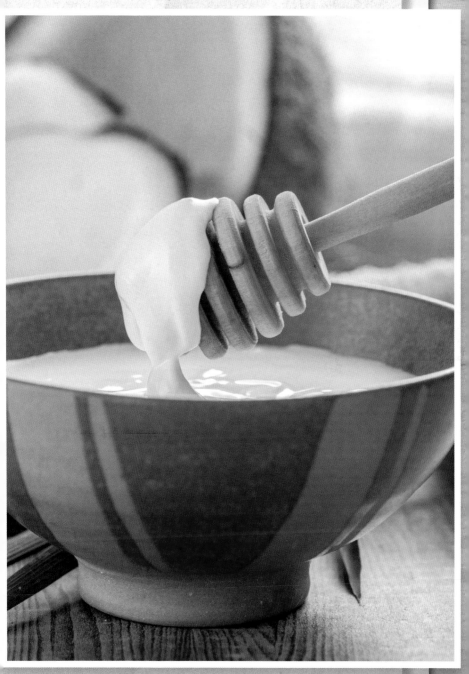

Apply coconut oil to soothe skin

WELLNESS

Coconut water has been consumed around the world as a hydrating drink that is high in nutrients and electrolytes, but its uses extend beyond that. Find out how coconut water can benefit your hair and skin as well as keep your body properly hydrated.

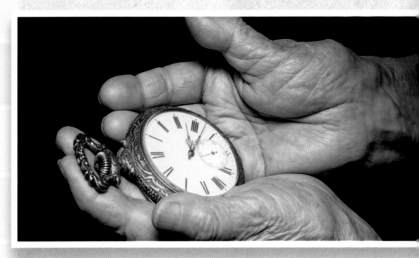

COMBAT AGING

Coconut water contains cytokines which help promote cell growth. This means that coconut water can help your skin repair faster as well as reduce any damage that has already taken place. Combine 1 tablespoon coconut water with 2 tablespoons plain yogurt and mix well. Using a soft brush, apply the mixture onto your face. Let it sit for 15 minutes and then rinse with cold water. As the lactic acid in yogurt is a gentle exfoliator, you should limit the use of this face mask to once or twice a week.

IMPROVE METABOLISM

Coconut water contains high levels of manganese, which is a crucial nutrient required for the proper metabolism of carbohydrates and fats into energy. Drinking coconut water can give your metabolism a boost.

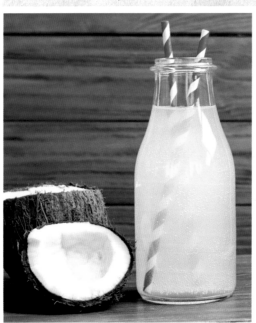

Drink coconut water to improve metabolism

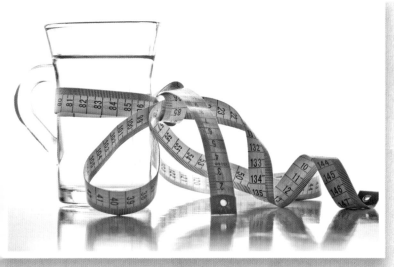

Coconut water can promote weight loss

AID DIGESTION

In order for your digestive system to function properly, you must ingest fiber. Coconut water is rich in fiber, making it a drink that is very beneficial for your digestive system. In fact, the water from a single coconut contains approximately 9% of the amount of fiber required by your body in a single day.

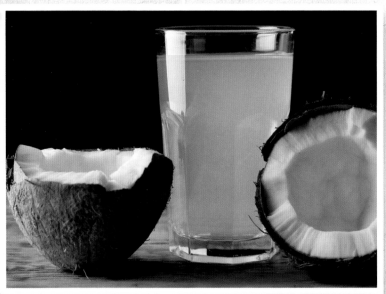

Coconut water contains elecrolytes

PREVENT DEHYDRATION

Dehydration occurs when the water content in your body drops too low, usually as a result of not drinking enough water or losing water through sweating or vomiting. Coconut water has high water content as well as being rich in nutrients—this can help replenish your body as you lose important salts and nutrients as well as water when you are dehydrated. Additionally, coconut water contains five key electrolytes: sodium, potassium, calcium, magnesium, and phosphorus, all of which are essential when treating dehydration.

WELLNESS

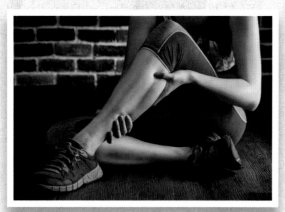

Coconut water combats dehydration and muscle fatigue

EASE LEG CRAMPS
Muscle cramps can occur due to a variety of reasons, including dehydration, potassium deficiency, and excessive exercise. Coconut water has high water content, which combats dehydration and muscle fatigue from exercising, as well as high levels of potassium and a number of crucial electrolytes. Coconut water can be a natural substitute for any energy drink.

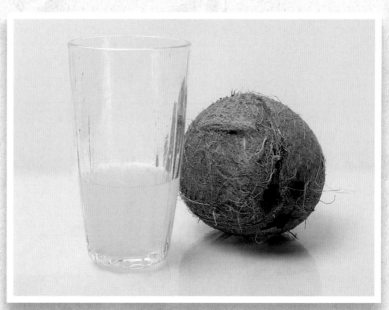

Coconut water is a good source of dietary fiber

AID WEIGHT LOSS
Coconut water has high water content, which can help make you feel full. Additionally, coconut water is a good source of dietary fiber. Fiber is not digested by your body; it stays in your system longer and helps to keep you feeling full, meaning you rarely feel hungry and eat less. However, it is important to remember that while coconut water is a good source of dietary fiber, it is also fairly high in sugar and should not be consumed in excess for that reason.

BOOST YOUR IMMUNITY

Coconut water contains 2.4mg of vitamin C in every 100 grams. Vitamin C is required by your body for the production of antibodies to fight off any foreign invasion. Coconut water also has natural antimicrobial peptides that are effective in fighting harmful bacteria.

FACE MASK

The most important element of good skin care is hydration; harsh soaps, pollution, and sun exposure can all dry your skin. Coconut water is a great moisturizer for your skin as it is lightweight and hydrates your skin without leaving it feeling greasy.

Coconut Water Face Mask

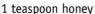

2 tablespoons coconut water
½ teaspoon fresh lemon juice
1 teaspoon honey

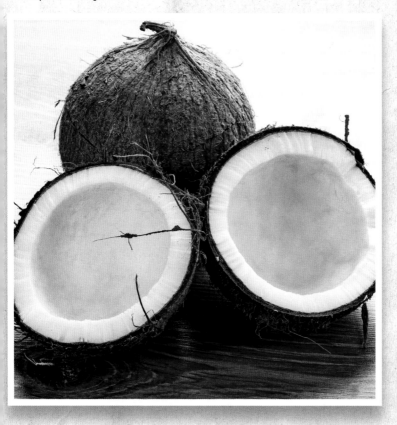

Combine the coconut water, lemon juice, and honey in a small bowl and stir well. Using a cotton ball or round, soak up the mixture and massage it into your skin using gentle, circular motions. Let the concoction sit for 30 minutes and then rinse with cold water. If you find that the level of lemon juice is too drying, try reducing to ¼ teaspoon. Alternatively, if you find that the level of honey is too rich for your skin type, you can lessen it or leave it out all together.

BEAUTY/PERSONAL

By incorporating coconut oil into your beauty routine, you can reap enormous benefits for your skin and hair. Many commercial face washes or soaps are harsh or drying and may actually be doing your skin more harm than good. Additionally, many shampoos contain ingredients that have been proven to damage your hair.

By using coconut oil in lieu of these products you can keep your skin and hair moisturized and clean in a natural way. From makeup remover to shaving cream, coconut oil can be used to give your beauty routine a healthy boost.

Coconut provides enormous natural benefits for your hair and skin

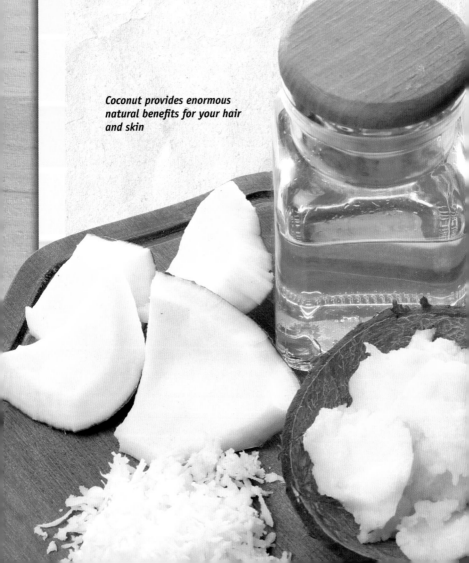

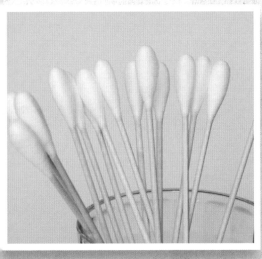

Use cotton buds to apply coconut oil

SPOT TREATMENT

Coconut oil consists of a number of medium-chain fatty acids such as lauric, capric, caproic, and caprylic acids. Each of these have strong antimicrobial effects and have been found to kill *Propionibacterium acnes*, which is one of the causes of acne. By applying coconut oil directly to the skin, its antibacterial properties can kill *P. acnes* as well as other bacteria that cause acne. Additionally, coconut oil can moisturize the skin; keeping the skin adequately moisturized will aide its ability to fight infection and heal, as well as prevent scarring.

While there are many benefits of applying coconut oil to your skin, it may not work for everyone. People with oily skin in particular may not benefit from applying coconut

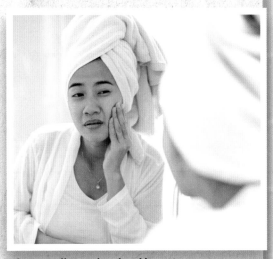

Coconut oil to moisturize skin

oil to their face, as coconut oil can clog pores. When applying coconut oil to your face, use a very thin layer. Additionally, if you like the process of using coconut oil on your skin but don't want it to clog your pores, you can apply it normally and then use a warm washcloth to gently wipe the excess oil off of your face.

BEAUTY/PERSONAL

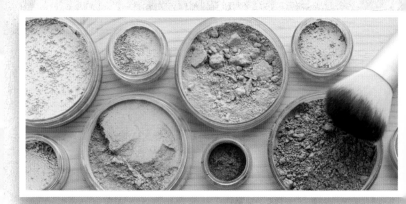

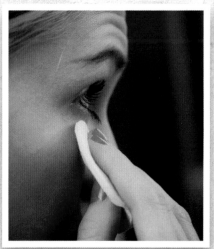

Use cotton rounds to remove makeup

MAKEUP REMOVER

Coconut oil can be used as a gentle, additive-free makeup remover that can handle everything from full-face foundation to waterproof mascara. Warm some coconut oil with your hands and gently rub into your skin in a circular motion. Use a cotton pad or round to remove the coconut oil and makeup with it. Repeat as needed and rinse once your makeup is removed.

HAIR CONDITIONER

Use coconut oil as a deep conditioner to give your hair the extra moisture it needs. Rub coconut oil into the ends of damp hair and let it sit for at least 30 minutes. For a more intense moisturizing effect, apply the coconut oil onto dry hair. Wash and style your hair as usual.

Tip: When applying the coconut oil, focus on the ends, as prolonged contact of the oil with your roots can make your hair greasy.

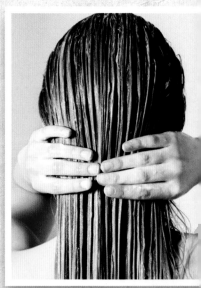

Condition hair with coconut oil

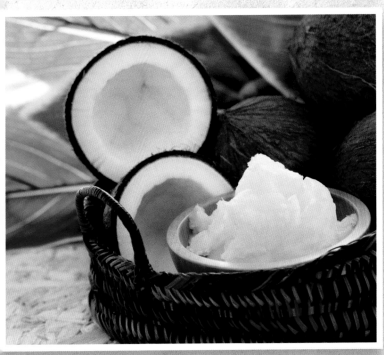

Coconut oil moisturizes skin

MASSAGE OIL

Coconut oil makes a wonderful massage oil due to its ability to penetrate skin and provide vitamin E. Coconut oil is easy to warm with your hands to make it the perfect consistency for a massage.

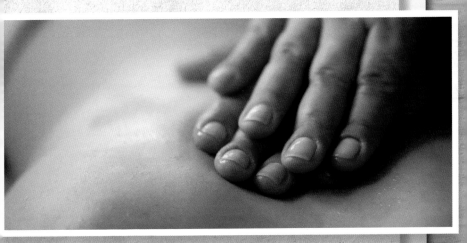

Give a massage with coconut oil

PERSONAL LUBRICANT

Coconut oil can be used as a personal lubricant as it contains no parabens, petroleum, glycerin, or other harmful additives. It is important to note, however, that coconut oil degrades latex, so is not safe to use with latex condoms or other products.

Tip: If you are planning on using any products that are made of latex, an organic water-based personal lubricant is a safer choice.

BEAUTY/PERSONAL

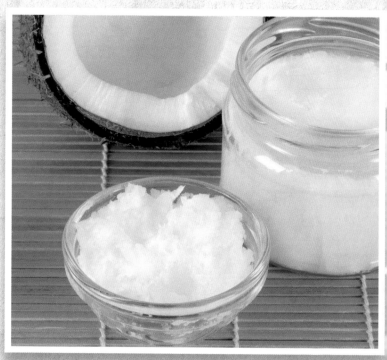

Coconut oil has many beauty uses

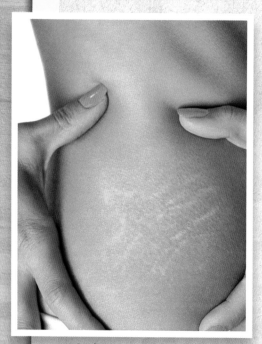

Apply coconut oil to stretch marks

MINIMIZE STRETCH MARKS

Stretch marks are scars that result from skin stretching too quickly or beyond its elastic capabilities and occur in men and women alike. While stretch marks are a natural and common experience, some people wish to prevent their occurrence and minimize their existing stretch marks. Coconut oil is an easy way to do that as it contains high levels of vitamin E, which can help repair damaged skin and keep the skin moisturized, reducing the production of more stretch marks.

While stretch marks are scars that cannot be eliminated through any topical means, the regular use of coconut oil can dramatically reduce the appearance of stretch marks as well as function as a preventative measure for further scarring.

ELIMINATE LICE

Lice are tiny parasites that invade hair shafts on the scalp and body. They are irritating to endure, difficult to remove, and are commonly a problem among children, although anyone is susceptible. Head lice reproduce very quickly, making it very difficult to eliminate the parasites. Many shampoos sold for the elimination of lice contain harmful ingredients. For a healthier approach, try these recipes.

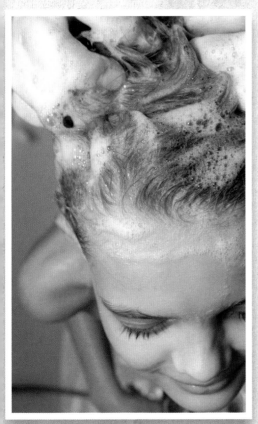

Lice Removal

Combine 1 teaspoon tea tree oil, 1 ounce child-friendly shampoo, and 3 tablespoons coconut oil. Apply the solution liberally throughout hair and onto scalp. Cover head with a shower cap and leave covered for at least 30 minutes. Rinse hair thoroughly with the hottest water you can tolerate. While hair is still wet, use a fine-toothed comb to remove any dead lice.

Use coconut oil to eradicate lice

Tip: Tea tree oil is a natural insecticide. By combining tea tree oil with coconut oil you can make an efficient lice remover.

Overnight Lice Removal

Rinse hair thoroughly with apple cider vinegar and allow it to dry. Follow up by completely saturating the hair and scalp with coconut oil. Cover head and hair with a shower cap and leave it on overnight, or at least 6 to 8 hours. Once time has passed, comb through hair and shampoo as usual. Repeat this process daily for 1 week to eradicate lice naturally.
Tip: Coconut oil will stop lice from moving and reproducing due to its lubricating nature.

BEAUTY/PERSONAL

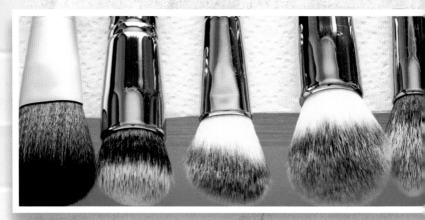

Keep your makeup brushes in good condition

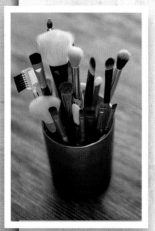

CLEAN MAKEUP BRUSHES

Keeping your makeup brushes clean is very important as dirty makeup brushes are a breeding ground for bacteria. Additionally, dirty brushes become dry and abrasive, meaning they are likely to irritate your skin. Regularly washing your makeup brushes ensures that your brushes maintain their quality for longer.

To make a DIY brush cleanser, combine 2 parts antibacterial soap and 1 part coconut oil. Simply apply the mixture to the brush you are cleaning and rub the bristles in a circular motion against your palm or a brush cleaning pad, then rinse with warm water. Repeat this process until the water runs clear and wring any excess water from the brush. To maintain their proper shape and to avoid damaging the handle of your brush, hang the brush upside down until completely dry.

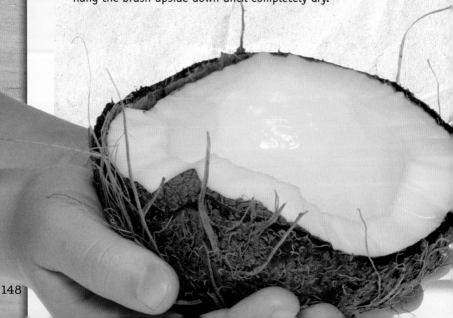

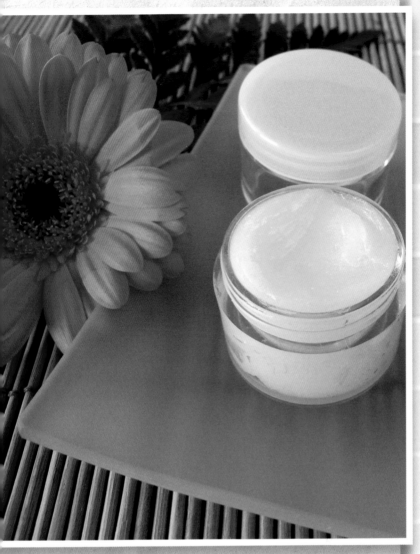

Travel-sized coconut oil

LIP BALM

Chapped and cracked lips can be annoying, painful, and unsightly. Many commercial sticks can actually worsen dry lips. For a natural solution, simply apply coconut oil to your lips regularly and be sure to drink plenty of water. For a convenient portable solution, just pack some coconut oil into a small jar or tin and apply to your lips throughout the day.

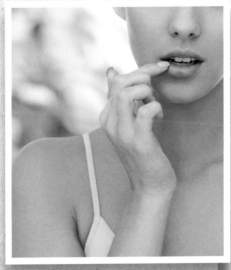

Apply to lips with your finger

BEAUTY/PERSONAL

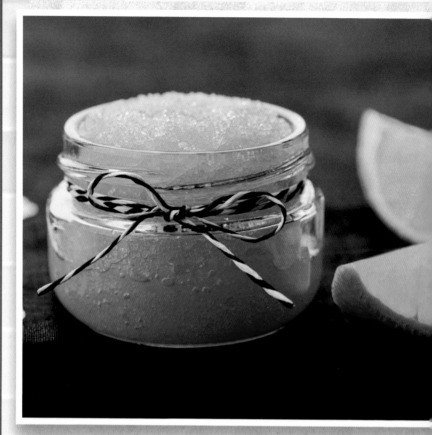

Make your own body scrub

BODY SCRUB

Follow these simple recipes to create a moisturizing, exfoliating body scrub. You'll save money by opting for these scrubs over store-bought alternatives and you'll benefit your body and the environment by using natural ingredients stored in reusable containers. Gently scrub your body with the mixture in the shower and rinse to reveal smooth, moisturized skin.

VERSATILE BODY SCRUB

Combine ¼–½ cup granulated sugar with ½ cup coconut oil. The amount of sugar will depend on how coarse you want your scrub to be and the type of sugar will determine the same: the larger the crystal, the more exfoliating the scrub. For a natural citrus scent, add 1 tablespoon citrus fruit zest. Depending on your preference, you can use lemon, grapefruit, lime, or orange. If you add citrus to your scrub, do not apply to your face, as it may irritate your skin and eyes.
Note: Be sure not to heat the coconut oil before combining ingredients, as it will melt the sugar.

HAND SCRUB

Combine ½ cup granulated sugar with ¼ cup coconut oil and mix thoroughly. This ration of sugar to coconut oil provides a much higher level of exfoliation and is therefore perfect for your hands. Try adding citrus zest or essential oils to your preference. **Note:** Adding essential oils to your scrub will ensure a longer shelf life than if you were to add citrus zest.

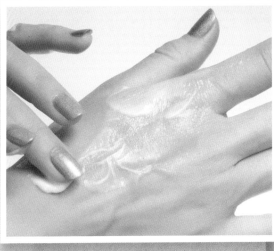

Use scrub to moisturize hands

SALT SCRUB

Combine 2 cups coconut oil with 1 cup Epsom salt and stir. Add essential oils or citrus zest to your preference to add scent. Store in a lidded jar.

Warning: Be careful when using any of these body scrubs in the shower as the coconut oil may leave your tub slippery. Particular care should be taken when applied to your feet.

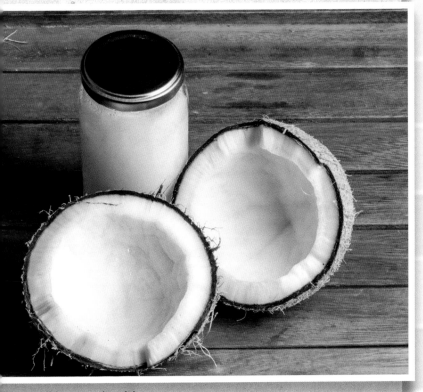

Coconut oil is very moisturizing

BEAUTY/PERSONAL

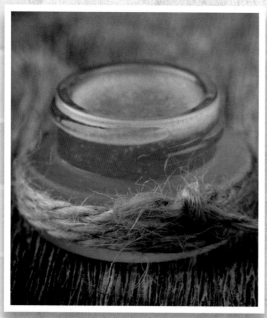

DIY lip scrub

LIP SCRUB

Combine 1 teaspoon coconut oil, 2 tablespoons sugar, and 1 tablespoon honey in a small bowl. Apply to the lips with a finger and gently rub in a circular motion to exfoliate any dead skin. This lip scrub can be made at need or you can make a larger amount and store it in a small jar or container. Try adding 1–2 drops of peppermint essential oil for a tingling sensation.

SHAVING CREAM

Many commercial shaving creams can dry your skin as you shave. Switch your old shaving cream out for your own coconut oil shaving cream for smooth, moisturized skin.

Coconut Oil Shaving Cream

¾ cup grated shea butter soap
¼ cup coconut oil
¼ cup aloe vera gel
¼ cup witch hazel

Tip: Be sure to use a witch hazel that does not contain alcohol.

Grate shea butter soap. Combine grated soap, coconut oil, and witch hazel into a small heat-safe bowl and place it in a saucepan or pot of water to create a double boiler. Heat the pan on a low flame until the soap melts, stirring occasionally. Once the mixture

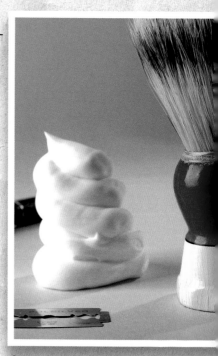

Create coconut oil shaving cream

has been thoroughly combined, carefully remove from the heat and add the aloe vera gel. You can add a few drops of your favorite essential oils at this stage if you wish. Combine the mixture well by hand or with an immersion blender. Once the mixture is room temperature, mix again to create a creamy consistency. Store your new shaving cream in a reusable squeeze tube or a lidded jar or container and apply with your fingers.

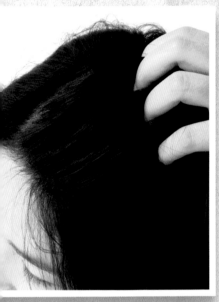

pply coconut oil to scalp

TREAT DANDRUFF

Often times, dandruff is the result of a dry scalp. Get right to the source of the problem by moisturizing your scalp nightly with coconut oil. Apply a light amount of coconut oil to your roots and gently massage, efficiently applying the oil and stimulating hair growth. Rinse after at least 1 hour or let sit overnight, then shampoo hair as usual.

Tip: If your hair gets too greasy from the coconut oil, reduce the frequency of this treatment.

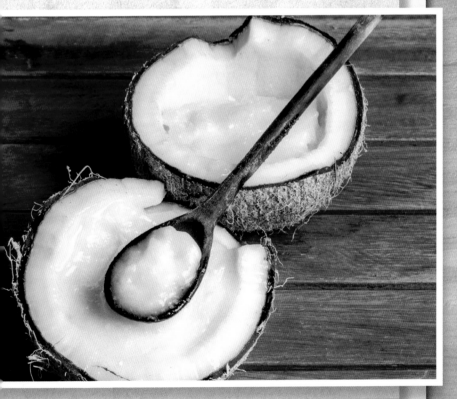

BEAUTY/PERSONAL

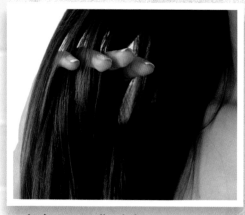

Apply coconut oil to hair

TAME FRIZZ

If you have frizzy hair, simply warm a dime-sized amount of coconut oil in your palms and smooth the ends of your hair to eliminate frizz and amplify shine. Be sure to rub the coconut oil over your entire hand to avoid any uneven coconut oil application.

CRACKED CUTICLES

Just as coconut oil can remedy cracked lips, it can do wonders for your cuticles. Apply coconut oil directly to the base of your nails to counter peeling skin and keep your nails healthy.

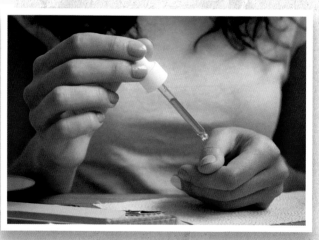

Keep your cuticles healthy

DEEP CONDITION

For healthy hair and ends, take a generous amount of coconut oil and warm it in your hands before applying it to your hair. Finger-comb the oil through dry hair for a pre-shower treatment and let it sit for at least 1 hour before shampooing and conditioning as usual.

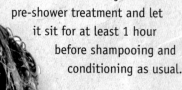

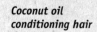

Coconut oil conditioning hair

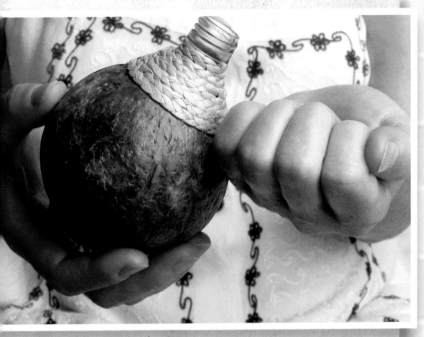

Pour coconut oil into your hand

BODY OIL

After a shower, apply a light layer of coconut oil to your skin for a moisturizing bonus and pat dry.

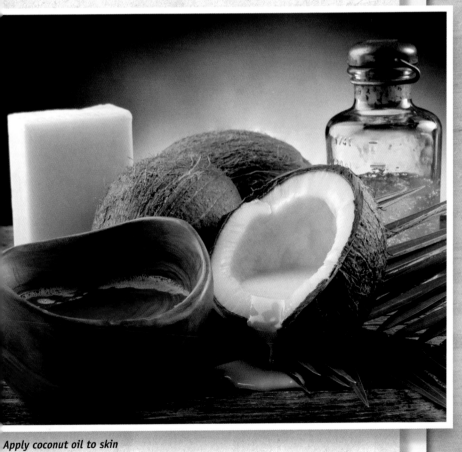

Apply coconut oil to skin

BEAUTY/PERSONAL

REDUCE ACNE

As coconut water possesses antibacterial properties, it can be used to combat acne. Make a natural toner by combining ½ cup coconut water with 1 teaspoon honey. Soak a cotton ball or round in the mixture and dab onto a clean, dry face. Let it sit for 10 minutes and gently wipe it away with a damp washcloth. Honey also possesses antibacterial and anti-inflammatory properties; the combination of honey and coconut water can reduce swelling and soothe your skin.

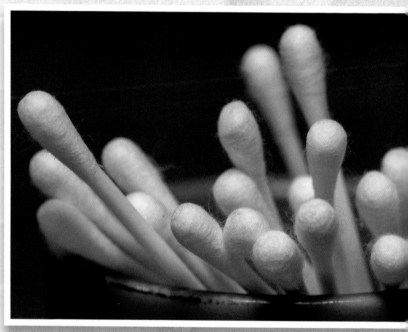

Use cotton buds to apply coconut water

Coconut milk contains high levels of iron, sodium, selenium, calcium, magnesium, and phosphorus, as well as vitamins B1, B3, B5, B6, C, and E. Your hair and skin both need many of these vitamins and nutrients to stay healthy and coconut milk can provide a solution.

STIMULATE HAIR GROWTH

Coconut water contains nutrients that can help your hair grow. As a lack of certain nutrients can stunt hair growth or cause hair to fall out, coconut water could be the natural solution to your hair problems. Simply massage ½ cup coconut water into your scalp regularly to aid hair growth. Massage the coconut water into your scalp with your fingers and let it sit overnight. In the morning, shampoo as normal. You can use this method up to every other day.

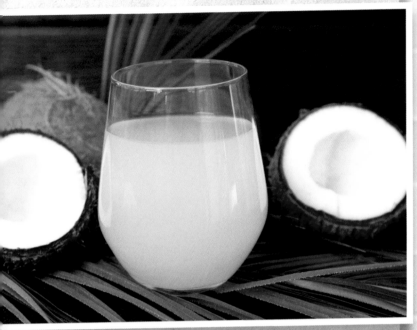

Coconut water contains nutrients that can help your hair grow

RESTORE DAMAGED HAIR

Coconut milk can be used as a tonic for an itchy, dry, and irritated scalp due to its excellent moisturising properties. Apply coconut milk to your scalp and massage gently for at least 5 minutes or so. Follow this process with a hot towel for a nourishing effect. This method is particularly beneficial for restoring dry, brittle, and damaged hair and split ends.

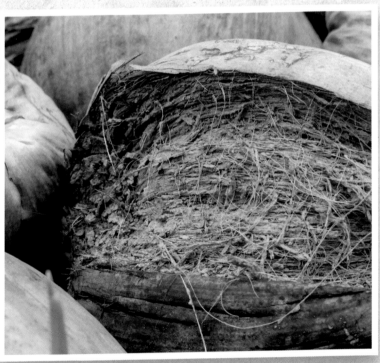

Coconut milk can be used as a tonic for an itchy, dry, and irritated scalp

BEAUTY/PERSONAL

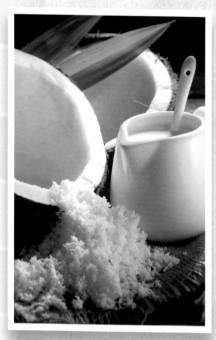

Shaved coconut and milk

CONDITION YOUR HAIR

Combine coconut milk with your regular shampoo in an equal-parts mixture to condition your hair while you clean it. Additionally, you can use coconut milk as a leave-in conditioner, which will add volume to your hair and make it less greasy.

MAKEUP REMOVER

To make a gentle makeup remover, combine 2 parts olive oil with 1 part coconut milk. Using a cotton pad or round, apply the mixture to your face and gently wipe your makeup away. Not only will it effortlessly remove your makeup, but it will leave your skin deeply nourished.

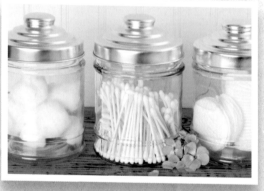

Condition hair with coconut

LEAVE-IN CONDITIONER

Coconut milk can be used to restore and detangle hair while promoting growth. Store coconut milk in a spray bottle and spray the ends of your hair to help brushing.

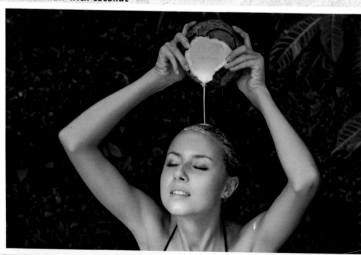

ACNE PREVENTION

The antibacterial properties of coconut milk make it a good natural cleanser for those with oily and acne prone skin. The fats in coconut milk do not clog pores, lowering the possibility of a breakout.

MOISTURIZE THE SKIN

Coconut milk has soothing properties, making it a great moisturizer. Apply coconut milk directly onto the skin and rub it in for 20–30 minutes to promote

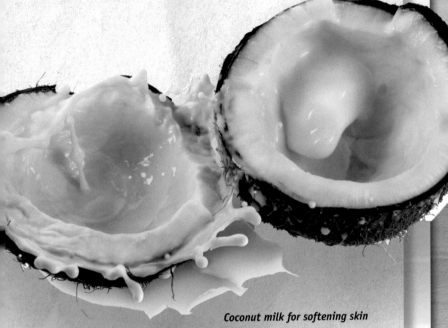

Coconut milk for softening skin

healthy skin and combat dryness. To add a moisturizing element to your bath, add 1 cup coconut milk to the water. Soak for about 15 minutes to help restore dry skin.

TREAT SKIN TROUBLE

The fatty acids in coconut milk can help treat dry and irritated skin caused by skin complains such as eczema, dermatitis, and psoriasis. Additionally, the antibacterial properties of coconut milk may help remove harmful bacteria.

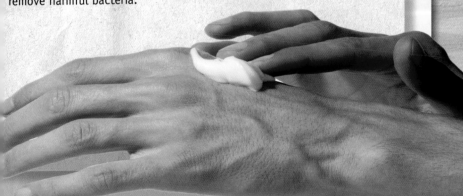

BEAUTY/PERSONAL

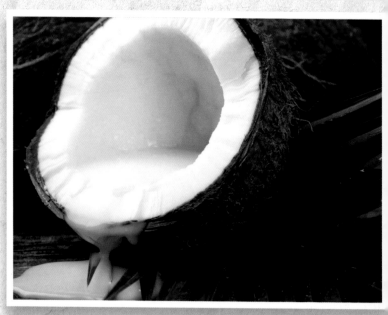

BODY SCRUB

Beauty aids with coconut milk

In a coffee grinder or food processor, grind ½ cup dry rice. Combine rice with ½ cup coconut milk, ¼ cup brown sugar, and 1½ tablespoons grated ginger in a small bowl. Stir until you have a thick, evenly-mixed paste. Apply this mixture over your entire body, rubbing in circular motions to exfoliate the skin. Rinse the mixture off in the shower to reveal moisturized skin.

PIÑA COLADA AGE SPOT MASK

Pineapple is a good choice for battling age spots and blotches; its high levels of vitamin C and the enzyme bromelain make it excellent for your skin. In a blender, combine ¼ cup chopped fresh pineapple with 1 tablespoon coconut milk and blend until smooth. Spread a thin layer of the mixture over clean, dry skin and let it sit for 5–10 minutes. Rinse with warm water and pat your face dry with a soft towel. The enzyme bromelain is a natural exfoliator, so be sure not to use this mask more than once a week.

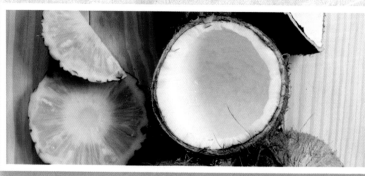

BODY WASH

In a clean, empty bottle, combine ¼ cup coconut milk with ½ cup liquid castile soap. Shake well to mix thoroughly. For best results, shake before each use. This natural, moisturizing body wash can also be used as face wash or shampoo.

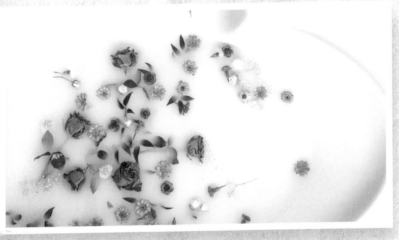

Luxurious Milk Bath Soak

MILK BATH SOAK

Combine 2 cups coconut milk and 1 tablespoon honey in a bowl. Take ½ cup old fashioned oats and grind them into a powder, then add to the coconut milk and honey. Once combined, add the mixture into your bath water and soak.

If you're preparing the bath soak for someone special, you can add flowers to give it a beautiful look.

> **WARNING!**
> Do not use oats if you are allergic to them. Some people with Celiac disease can be sensitive to them as well.

SUGAR SCRUB

For a healthy homemade body scrub, combine ½ cup coconut milk with ½ cup granulated sugar. For an added moisturizing bonus, add 1–2 teaspoons coconut oil. Stir well, then apply the mixture to the skin using your hands, rubbing in circular motions to thoroughly exfoliate the skin.

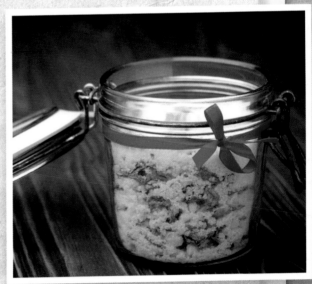

Store all scrubs in lidded jars

161

HOME

So many commercial cleaning products contain ingredients that can be harmful for your children and pets, as well as being expensive. For a natural way to keep your home clean and healthy, try using coconut oil. As coconut oil has high levels of saturated fat, it is slow to oxidize and therefore will keep longer than other oils.

Coconut oil is a popular ingredient in kitchens and bathrooms, as it can be used for anything from seasoning your cast iron to making soap. As it is relatively inexpensive, coconut oil is an affordable product that you can use to keep your home in good shape.

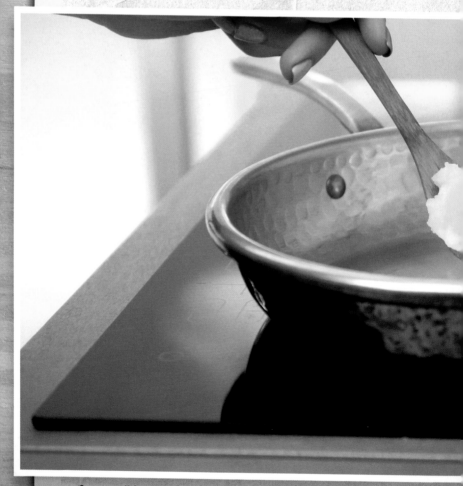

Coconut oil is a healthy cooking option

HEALTHY COOKING OIL

Coconut oil is an excellent choice for cooking. Coconut oil differs from the majority of other cooking oils as it contains a unique composition of fatty acids. While, like all oils, the fatty acids in coconut oil are about 90% saturated, coconut oil has a high content of saturated fat lauric acid, which accounts for approximately 40% of its total fat content. Because of this, coconut oil is highly resistant to oxidation at high heat, making it a suitable option for medium and high-heat cooking methods.

As coconut oil is rich in lauric acid, a unique type of saturated fat, it seems that moderate consumption of coconut oil can improve the levels of lipids circulating in the blood, potentially reducing the risk of heart disease. Additionally, studies have associated an increase in high-density lipoprotein (HDL) cholesterol, relative to total cholesterol, with a reduced risk of heart disease. Coconut oil significantly increases HDL cholesterol compared to the cooking alternatives of extra-virgin olive oil and butter.

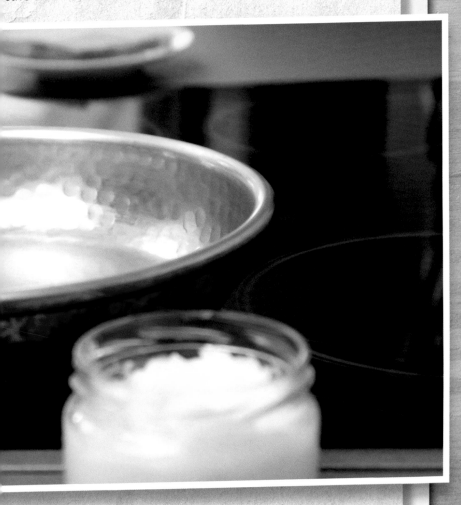

HOME

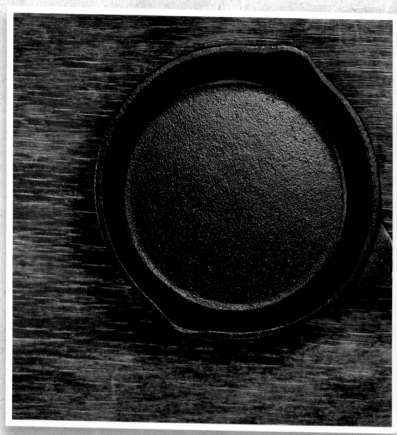

Coconut oil adds a minimal amount of fat to the pan.

SEASON CAST IRON PANS

A good-quality cast iron skillet should be a kitchen staple of every home. When properly cared for, cast iron skillets can last a lifetime, unlike other non-stick pans that can be damaged easily or corrode over time. Additionally, cast iron pans can transfer from the stove top into the oven and vice versa without a hitch, as they can withstand temperatures well above what is considered safe for traditional nonstick pans. Cast iron pans, with proper use, can function as a nonstick pan with superior durability and even heating. Proper cast iron care involves proper cleaning and regular seasoning. Luckily, seasoning your cast iron skillet or pan is very simple.

Cast iron skillet

By seasoning your cast iron skillet, you are creating a protective coating that gives the skillet its nonstick properties. While you can use a variety of oils to season your cast iron, coconut oil is a great option as it does not add an excessive amount of fat to the pan.

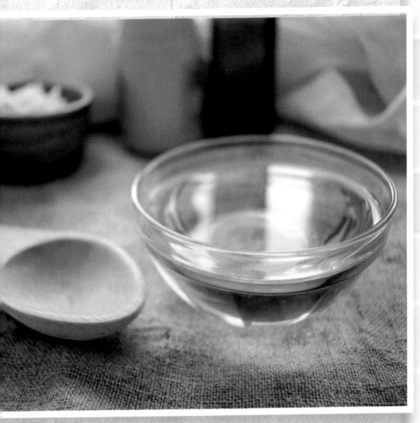

Use coconut oil for seasoning your cast iron pans

In order to properly season your cast iron, follow these steps. After you have used your cast iron, be sure to clean it properly. You shouldn't use dish soap on a cast iron and it should never go in the dishwasher, as it will remove the hard-earned seasoning from your

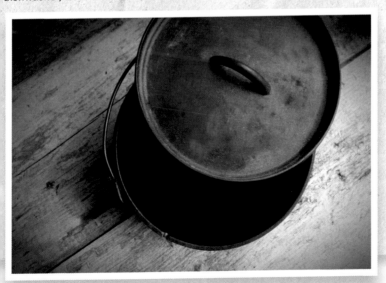

HOME

skillet and can potentially be absorbed into the surface of the pan. Instead, use a scouring brush, coarse salt, and the hottest water you can stand to remove any excess grime or food remnants. The best time to clean your cast iron is while it's still warm from cooking. Once done, completely dry your pan with a paper towel or cloth and put it on the stove over low heat to remove any surface water from the pan before continuing onto the next step of seasoning.

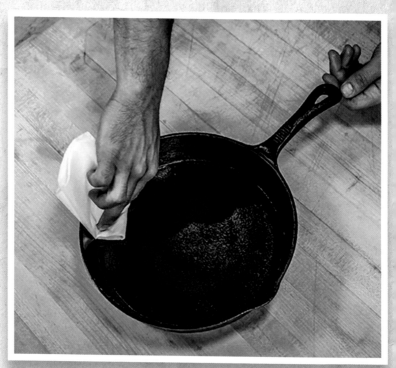

Dry your pan with a paper towel or cloth

Once your pan is completely dry and cool enough to handle, take a paper towel or soft cloth and apply a thin coat of coconut oil over the entire surface of the skillet, including the handle and underside of the pan. While you don't cook with the outside of your skillet, seasoning the entire surface will prevent any rust from developing. With a clean paper towel or cloth, rub off all excess oil and work the oil into the surface of the skillet. It seems counterintuitive, but you want to get it to the point where the pan looks like there is no oil left on the surface. This will give you the perfect amount of oil before you heat it.

Once the pan has been coated in oil, place the cast iron into the oven face down. Set your oven to its highest temperature, between 400–500°F and let the pan preheat with the oven. Once your oven reaches temperature, heat for at least 30 minutes; it is important to bring the oil above its smoke point. This will initiate the release of free

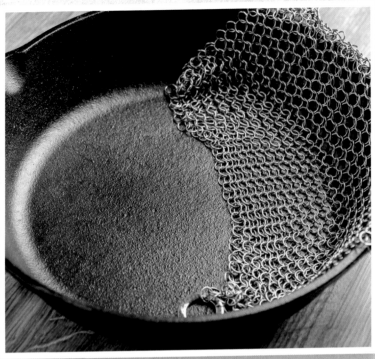

Using a chain mail "cloth" is another good way to clean your cast iron pans

radicals and polymerization, creating that nonstick sheen that cast iron is famous for. Additionally, if the oil does not go above its smoke point, it can go rancid and effect the flavor and safety of your meals.

After the cast iron has been at temperature for the alloted time, turn your oven off and leave the pan in the oven while it cools. After 2 hours, it will be cool enough to handle. If your cast iron is new, it may not look like much has happened— this is normal. Simply repeat the process and enjoy your properly seasoned cast iron skillet.

WARNING!

While bringing oil past its smoke point is good for seasoning cast iron, it's bad for you! Do not eat food that has been cooked in oil that smokes.

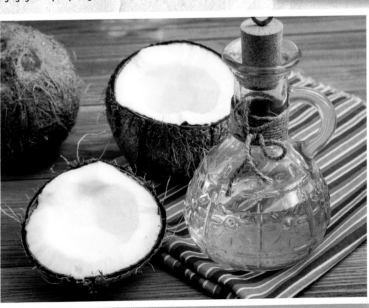

HOME

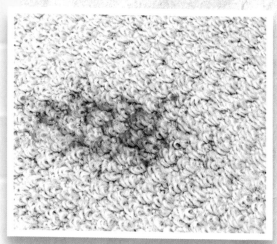

Remove stains from carpet

STAIN REMOVER

Coconut oil can be used as an effective stain remover in carpets and upholstery. By switching from commercial stain removers to coconut oil, you can keep your home looking clean without any harmful ingredients.

To remove an ink or crayon stain from your carpet or upholstery, blot some coconut oil into the spot to loosen the stain. For a boost, mix in baking soda and lightly rub the area with a soft toothbrush in circular motions.

To remove ink stains from plastic or vinyl, apply small amounts of coconut oil into the stain and buff in circular motions using a rag until the stain is removed.

Tip: Coconut oil can also be used to safely remove any residue left by stickers from plastic, glass, wood, and any other hard surface.

FURNITURE POLISH

Use coconut oil as a natural wood polish to prolong life and prevent cracking. Commercial furniture polish contain ingredients such as phenol and nitrobenzene, both of which have been proven to have damaging effects on your body.

To make a natural, affordable, and effective furniture polish, combine ½ cup coconut oil with ¼ cup fresh lemon juice

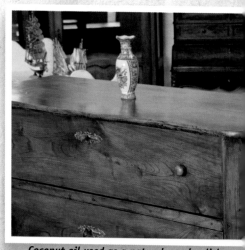

Coconut oil used as a natural wood polish

in glass and stir. Using a soft polishing cloth, apply the mixture to any wooden surfaces in your home. Work with the grain to initially apply the polish and then buff the mixture into the surface.

Tip: Be sure to dust any wooden surfaces before applying your natural polish!

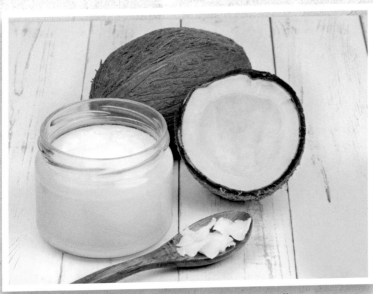

Coconut oil to remove gum

REMOVE GUM

If you have gum stuck in your hair, apply a generous amount of coconut oil directly to the gum and let it sit for a minute or two before slowly sliding the gum out of your hair. Coconut oil is more pleasant to work with than peanut butter and there's the added bonus of some moisturizing treatment for your ends.

FIX A CAUGHT ZIPPER

To unstick a caught zipper, apply some coconut oil along the length of both sides of the zipper using a cotton ball, cotton round, or your fingers. Gently work zipper until free.

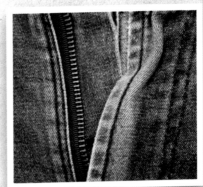

Apply coconut oil to a stuck zipper

PREVENT DUST

To prevent dust accumulation on surfaces around your home, try coconut oil. Simply apply a small amount of coconut oil to any wooden, plastic, or cement surfaces using a paper towel or soft cloth. Let the oil dry and then wipe off any excess with a clean towel.

Coconut oil can prevent dust

HOME

SHINE SHOES

Coconut oil can function as an excellent leather shoe conditioner. To properly maintain your shoes, be sure to keep your boots dry. Avoid wearing the same pair of shoes every day to give them time to air out between wears and make sure your socks are fresh. Before conditioning your shoes, make sure that they are clean. Dampen a cloth with water and wipe the surface of the shoe to ensure that the boot is clean before you condition to avoid trapping dirt and causing the boots to wear down faster. You can also use a horsehair brush to brush your boots.

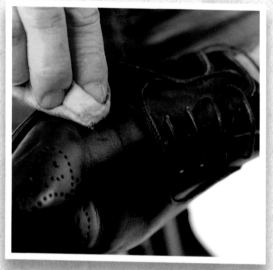

Use a rag to apply coconut oil

Once your shoes are clean and dry, apply a thin, even coat of liquid coconut oil onto the boots using your hands or a clean paper towel or cloth. Once the oil has been evenly applied to the boots, use a fresh towel or cloth to remove any excess oil.

Conditioning with coconut oil is most effective when the oil is in liquid form. As coconut oil has a melting point of 76°F, you can melt the oil using your hands. You should condition your leather shoes every 4–8 months. Cleaning can be done more regularly, after every 5 wears or so.

RUST REDUCER

Rust is an annoying problem that can turn up anywhere. Over time, rust will damage a metallic object until it is unusable. Many commercial solutions made to combat rust contain toxic ingredients. Coconut oil is one of the best natural rust removers that will safely remove rust from your household objects and protect the environment from harmful toxins, as well as being much more inexpensive. You can apply coconut oil directly to the surface either alone or in combination with other kitchen staples.

For rusted bathroom taps or faucets, sprinkle a small amount of baking soda over the affected areas. Follow with a washcloth dipped in coconut oil and scrub the areas where you have applied the baking soda. For an extra boost, try using white vinegar rather than baking soda for the initial application and then switch to baking soda.

For a homemade rust remover you can prepare, combine 1 tablespoon coconut oil with ½ teaspoon lemon juice in a small bowl. Apply this mixture to any affected areas using a paintbrush.

Tip: Do a patch test on your furniture in an unobtrusive area to ensure that no damage will occur.

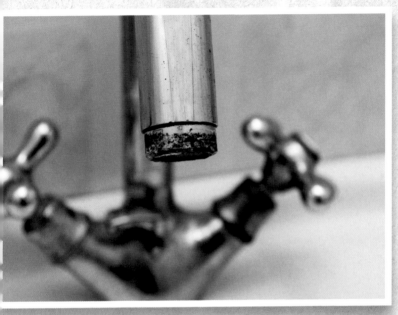

Remove rust from faucets

For a general rust remover, simply apply a thin layer of coconut oil to the rusty item using a paper towel or clean cloth. Set the item aside for at least 1 hour to ensure best results. Rinse the object in warm water until clean, then dry.

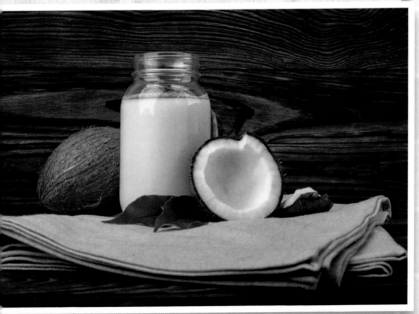

HOME

HEALTHY HAND SOAP

Making your own hand soap using coconut oil is simple and cost effective. Many hand soaps contain ingredients that will dry your skin. By using coconut oil you can create a soap that has plenty of lather and will properly clean and moisturize your hands.

Five-minute Hand Soap

2 tablespoons castile soap
2 teaspoons fractionated coconut oil
5–10 drops tea tree or other essential oil (optional)

For this hand soap you will need a clean, empty hand soap dispenser. Remove the pump, and add castile soap, fractionated coconut oil, and any tea tree or other essential oils, if desired. Fill the bottle the rest of the way with water, making sure to leave room for the pump. Shake well to combine the ingredients. For best results, shake well before each use.
Tip: Fractionated coconut oil has had the long-chain fatty acids removed through hydrolysis and steam distillation, making the oil liquid at room temperature and extending the product's shelf life. Fractionated coconut oil is completely soluble with other oils, making it a popular choice for skin products as it maintains its moisturizing capabilities.

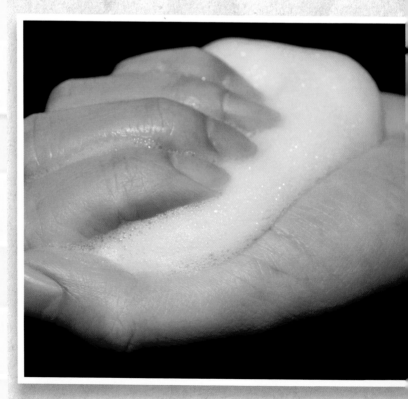

Gallon of Hand Soap

4 cups coconut oil
8.59 ounces potassium
hydroxide flakes (KOH)
2¼ cups water
1 cup glycerin

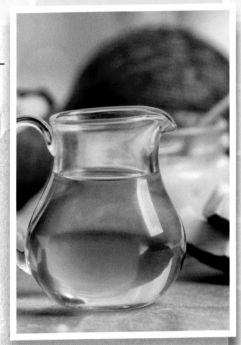

For this hand soap you will need a slow cooker, an immersion blender, and an electric scale. In your crockpot, melt coconut oil over a low heat. In a separate bowl, mix water and glycerin. In a third bowl, measure out potassium hydroxide flakes, then pour into the water and glycerin mixture. Mix well until the potassium hydroxide flakes are properly dissolved.

Coconut oil is a common ingredient found in many soaps

Once dissolved, pour this mixture into the coconut oil and slowly combine while mixing. Switch to the immersion blender and blend ingredients together with the slow cooker still on low heat. After a few minutes of blending, the mixture should start to look grainy and thicken. If the mixture becomes too thick for the immersion blender, switch to a wooden spoon and mix by hand. The mixing process should take between 3–4 hours with the mixture becoming thicker and more translucent. After the correct amount of time, remove a small amount of soap paste and dissolve it in water; if the liquid is cloudy, you will need to continue cooking the soap. If it is clear, your soap paste is done.

Once your soap paste is finished, you can remove it from the slow cooker and store it for when you want to dilute it into hand soap. It's a good idea not to dilute all of your soap at once, as adding water will shorten its shelf life. To dilute your soap paste, combine equal parts soap paste and water in a slow cooker and stir well. If your slow cooker is still hot from your soap making, you can simply turn it off and use the remaining heat to dilute your soap. If it is not, you can turn the heat to low for several hours. You can check on it and stir occasionally; after a while you will have clear soap.

This soap recipe is a little more time consuming, but the outcome is much more soap that can be used for washing your hands as well as general house cleaning.

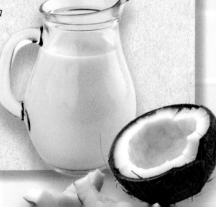

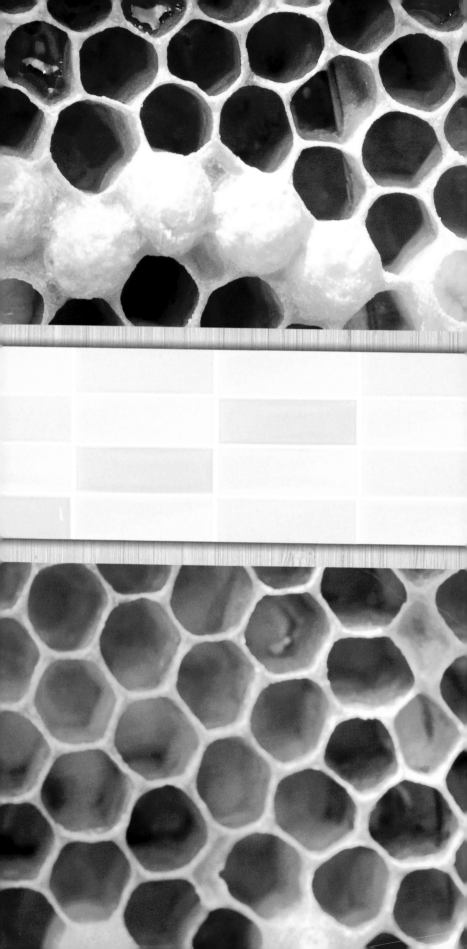

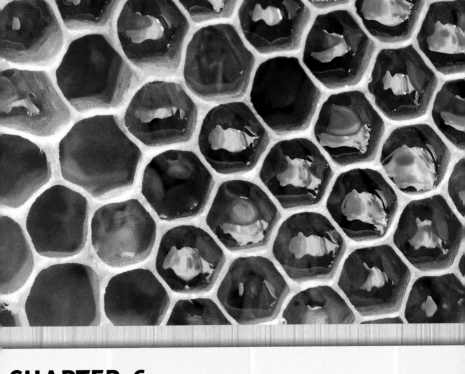

CHAPTER 6

HONEY

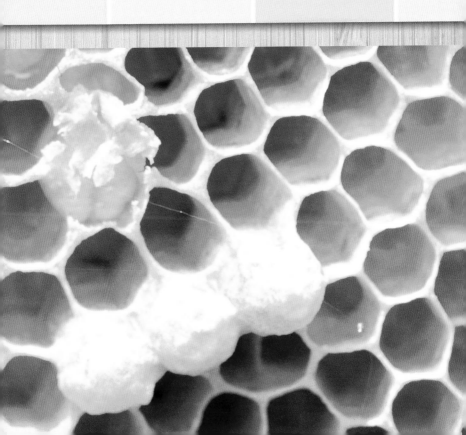

HONEY USES

While honey is delicious in tea or drizzled over cereal, it is also a wonderful source of wellness. Honey has a variety of benefits that can improve your health and your beauty routine. Additionally, beeswax, which is a byproduct of honey, is an incredibly useful item to use around the house; you can use it to polish furniture, moisturize your skin, and even make your own perfume.
Find out how you can use this sweet substance.

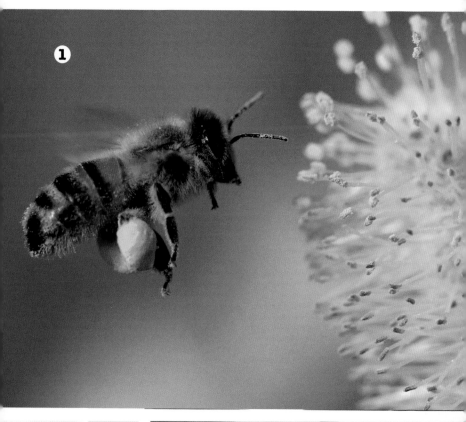

1 Honey bee
2 Natural beeswax soap
3 Honey, ginger, and lemon tea
4 Honey

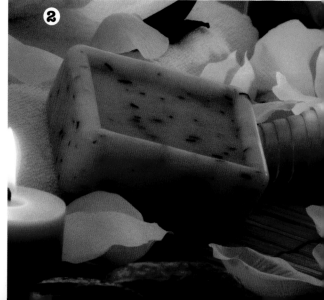

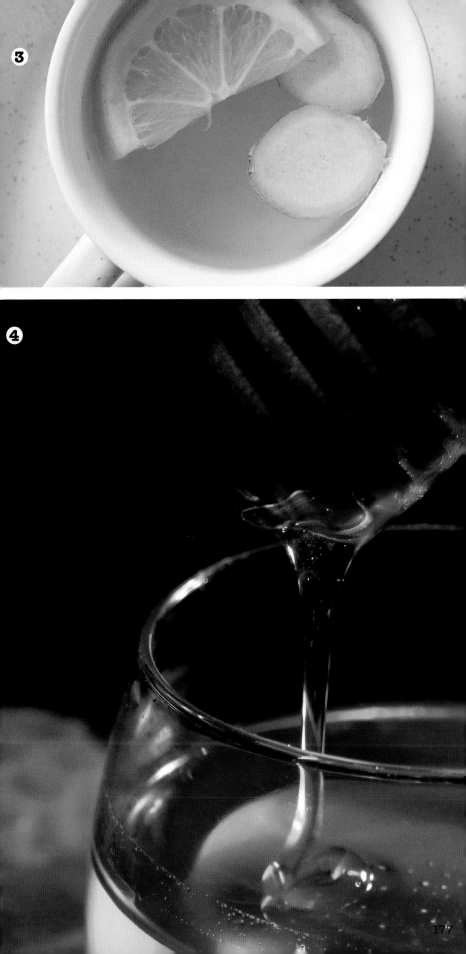

WELLNESS

For centuries, honey has been used as a natural healer. Composed of mostly sugar and water, honey is known for its antibacterial properties, particularly manuka honey, which is sourced in New Zealand and has the most effective antibacterial and anti-inflammatory properties. Honey also contains a number of other substances, including nutrients, enzymes, and antioxidants.

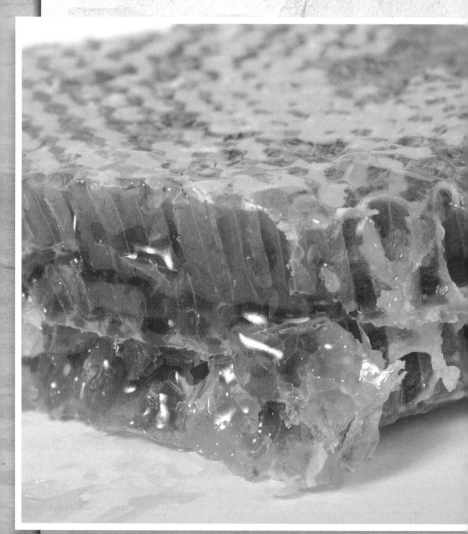

While honey is already a staple of most kitchen cupboards, it may be owed a place in your medical cabinet as well.

HELP HEAL CUTS

Honey naturally has antibacterial properties. Honey—specifically raw manuka honey, which is a honey found in New Zealand—can be very effective in speeding up the healing of small cuts. If you have a cut, apply honey and cover the affected area to increase the healing process. Be sure to consult a physician if you are unsure of whether a cut is insignificant.

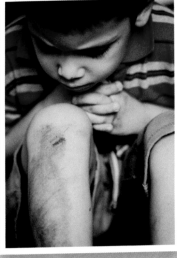

Honey helps cuts heal

FIGHT A COLD

Cough syrup is often filled with ingredients that can be damaging to your body. For a natural cough syrup, try making your own honey-based recipe.

Honey Cough Syrup

1 quart water
¼ cup minced ginger
1 tablespoon cinnamon
¼ cup fresh lemon juice
1 cup honey

In a medium saucepan, combine water, ginger, and cinnamon. Bring mixture to a boil and reduce to a simmer; let the saucepan simmer until the volume is reduced by half. Remove from heat and pour mixture through a fine mesh strainer or cheesecloth to remove any ginger particles. While the liquid is still warm, add lemon juice and honey and stir well. Store in an airtight container. This mixture can be stored in the refrigerator for up to two months. To combat cough in adults, consume 1 tablespoon. For children, 1 teaspoon will be sufficient.

WARNING!
You should never give honey to a child under a year old, as honey can, very occasionally, contain a spore of a bacterium called *Clostridium botulinum*, which can cause a form of food poisoning (botulism) in babies.

REDUCE ACID REFLUX

Almost 20 percent of Americans regularly deal with acid reflux symptoms. While there are many over-the-counter options, there are several natural options available. 1 tablespoon honey, taken daily, can be very effective at countering acid reflux symptoms. Honey is rich in antioxidants, which can help protect your body from cell damage caused by free radicals. Additionally, honey has a number of antibacterial and antiviral properties, meaning that raw, organic honey can kill bacteria and fungus that may be contributing to acid reflux. The texture of honey can also coat the esophagus and lining of the stomach, which can contribute to longer-lasting relief.

WELLNESS

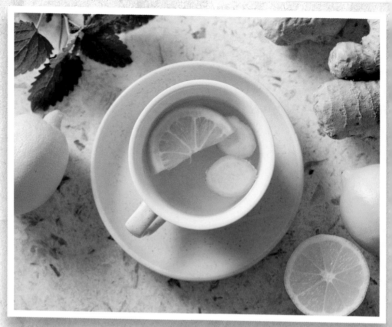

Soothe a sore throat with honey

SOOTHING TEA

If you have a cold, try making honey tea to alleviate your symptoms. In a teapot, pour 1½ cups boiling water over ½ tablespoon grated ginger. Let the ginger steep for at least 15 minutes before adding 1–2 tablespoons honey and ¼ cup fresh lemon juice. Stir well and serve immediately to soothe sore throats, congestion, and upset stomach symptoms.

COUGH DROPS

For a persistent cough, try making your own cough drops with honey and herbs.

Honey Cough Drops

½ cup honey
2 tablespoons fresh lemon juice
1 teaspoon fresh ginger, grated
Powdered sugar, cornstarch, or arrowroot powder

In a deep, medium-sized saucepan, combine honey, lemon juice, and ginger and mix well. Heat at medium-low heat until boiling. Stir often to prevent burning. If stirring causes the mixture to foam, remove from heat until the foam subsides, then return to heat. Using a candy thermometer, check the mixture regularly until it reaches 300°F. Remove mixture from heat and allow to cool until it thickens slightly. At this point, you can either pour the mixture into candy molds or simply drop 1 teaspoon worth of the mixture onto parchment paper or a silicone mat. Allow the mixture to cool until the cough drops are firm. Once the drops are cooled, toss them in powdered sugar, cornstarch, or arrowroot powder to prevent the drops from sticking together. Store your new cough drops in a closed container at room temperature or in the refrigerator during the summer months.

For an herbal boost, try this recipe:

Honey and Herb Drops

1 cup honey
1 cup strong, herbal tea
Powdered sugar, cornstarch, or arrowroot powder

In a bowl or saucepan, pour 1½ cups boiling water over herbal tea of your choice. Let the tea steep for at least 20 minutes before straining. In a small, deep saucepan, combine your herbal tea with 1 cup honey. For best results, a saucepan with a thick bottom should be used. Attach a candy thermometer to your saucepan and, over medium-low heat, let the mixture come to a boil and then simmer, stirring frequently, until the temperature reaches 300°F. Once this temperature has been reached, let the mixture cool until it begins to harden, then pour into candy molds or scoop 1 teaspoon of mixture at a time onto a parchment paper or silicone sheet. Once the drops are completely cool, toss them in the powdering agent of your choice and store in a closed container.

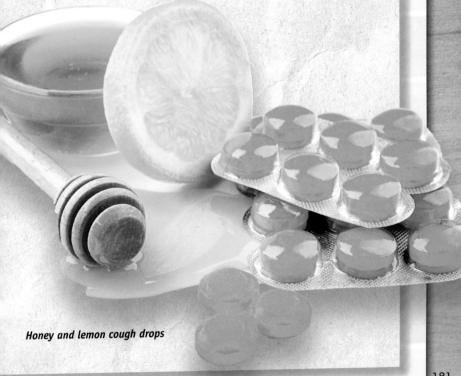

Honey and lemon cough drops

WELLNESS

SLEEP AID

If you have trouble sleeping, honey can make for a simple, effective sleep aid. If you are waking up in the middle of the night, it is possible that your blood sugar spiked, which will lead to interrupted sleep cycles. Before going to bed, take 1 teaspoon of raw, organic honey combined with ½ teaspoon salt.

solvency... The economy has entered a downturn, and unemployment and inflation can be expected to increase.

insolvent /ɪnsɒlvənt/. A person or organization that is **insolvent** does not have enough money to pay their debts; a formal word. *Two years later the bank was declared insolvent.*

insomnia /ɪnsɒmnɪə/. Someone suffering from **insomnia** finds it difficult to sleep.

insomniac /ɪnsɒmnɪæk/ **insomniacs.** An insomniac is a person who finds it difficult to sleep.

insouciance /ɪnsuːsɪəns/. **Insouciance** is the lack of concern shown by someone about something which they might be expected to take more seriously; a formal word. *He replied with apparent insouciance, 'So what?'*

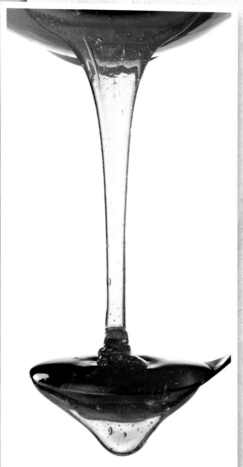

Honey can improve your sleep

BURN BALM

Honey is antibacterial and can soothe your skin. If you have a small burn, apply some honey to the area to reduce discomfort and improve healing time. It is important to note that anything more than a small, first-degree burn should not be initially treated with honey. If you are unsure of the severity of a burn, consult a physician.

CHAPPED LIPS

If you have chapped lips, try applying honey directly to the lips and let it sit for a moisturizing effect. For very chapped lips, try using a coconut oil sugar scrub (as seen on page 152) and follow up with honey.

GUT HEALTH

Honey is anti-inflammatory and antimicrobial. Consuming honey can regulate bacteria in the gut and improve your general gut health. Dilute 1 teaspoon honey in water to benefit from these effects. For best results, try manuka honey or the darkest honey available.

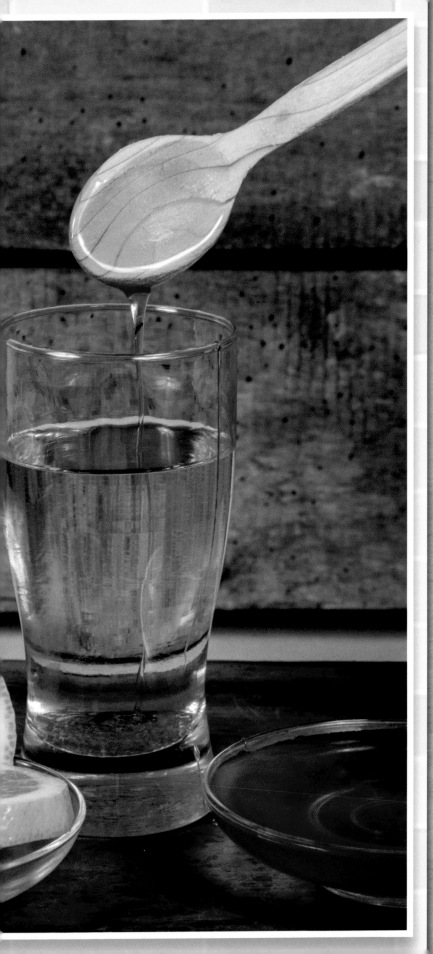

183

WELLNESS

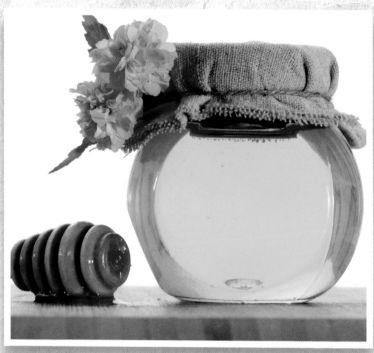

Use honey to lower cholesterol

LOWER CHOLESTEROL

In some studies, honey has been shown to lower cholesterol. Specifically, honey has been shown to reduce C-reactive protein, a marker of inflammation; LDL cholesterol; triglycerides; and homocysteine, a blood marker associated with disease. Additionally, honey has been shown to raise HDL cholesterol. While honey does contain these beneficial properties, honey is high in sugar and fructose, and has been shown to increase HbA1c, which is a marker of blood glucose levels.

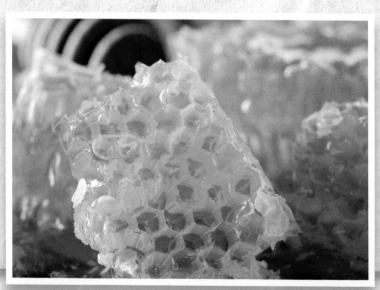

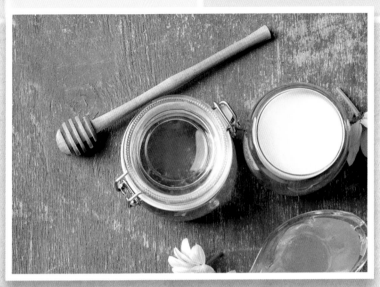

Honey is high in potassium

RELIEVE NAUSEA

Honey has many properties that can treat nausea very effectively. Honey exhibits antibacterial and antimicrobial properties that can help your gut counter any microbes causing any intestinal issues. Additionally, honey is enriched with enzymes that can help with proper digestion and relieve nausea. The high levels of potassium contained in honey can ease nausea and the coating quality of honey can soothe the stomach lining and esophagus to eliminate irritation from stomach acid.

The most effective method is to consume 2 teaspoons raw, organic honey 2–3 times daily. For best results, manuka honey is the best option. For an extra boost, try adding 1 teaspoon fresh lemon juice to your water and honey mixture. Additionally, you can try adding honey and fresh lemon juice to ginger tea, as ginger can also help with countering nausea.

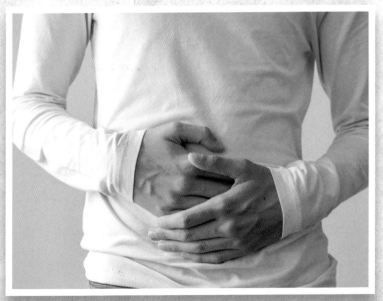

Honey can help figh nausea

BEAUTY/PERSONAL

Not only is honey excellent for your hair and skin, but most beauty treatments using honey are super simple. Honey's natural antibacterial properties and high levels of antioxidants will help keep your skin's glow and your hair's shine.

Honey can help moisturize, fight bacteria, and reverse the effects of aging. Raw, organic honey is best for your hair and skin as it contains more active phytonutrient antioxidants and enzymes. You can easily create at-home remedies that deliver on antioxidants, antimicrobial agents, and moisture for buzz-worthy results.

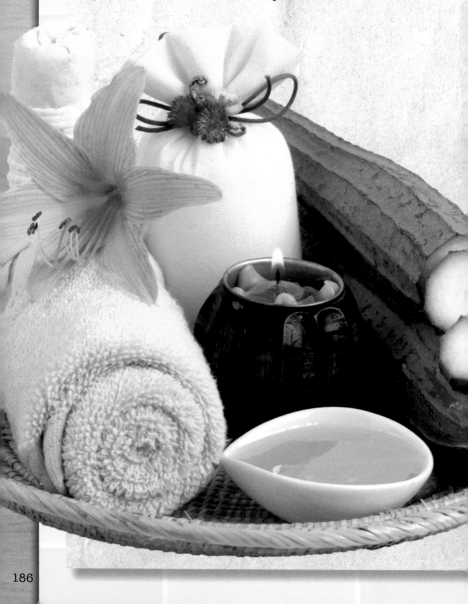

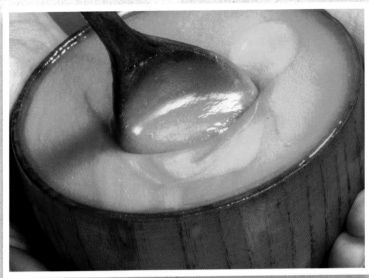

Honey and lemon face wash

FACE WASH

Honey is naturally antibiotic and is therefore an excellent, natural way to cleanse your skin. Simply place a small amount of raw, organic honey in your hands and massage the honey into your skin in circular motions.

For a deep pore cleanse, let the honey sit for up to 15 minutes before washing your face with warm water. Pat your face dry with a clean towel and enjoy soft, clean skin.

For easier application, try making a mixture of one part coconut oil and one part honey for a balmy texture that will glide over your skin effortlessly.

If you have oily skin, try adding a pinch of cinnamon to the honey before massaging it onto your face. Be sure to do a small test patch first to ensure that you have no adverse reaction to the cinnamon.

For age spots or discoloration, add 1 teaspoon of fresh lemon juice to the honey in a small bowl before applying to the skin to lighten dark spots and clean pores. Rinse thoroughly.

SHAMPOO

For extra-silky hair, try washing your hair with raw honey. For this method, simply massage a small amount of honey into the scalp and hair. Alternatively, you can mix 1 teaspoon raw, organic honey with a dime-sized amount of your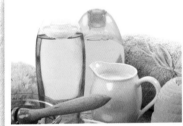

Honey and shampoo

favorite shampoo. Rinse your hair thoroughly with warm water. The humectant nature of honey helps to regulate and retain moisture in your hair while strengthening hair follicles.

BEAUTY/PERSONAL

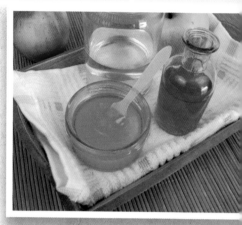

HAIR CONDITIONER

Many commercial hair conditioners contain sodium lauryl sulfate, which is a detergent and surfactant that creates a lather in many products such as shampoo and toothpaste (as well as engine degreaser and industrial strength detergents). While it is

Use honey to shine and soften hair

inexpensive and effective, it is a skin irritant and is also very drying. Products containing sodium lauryl sulfate will strip your hair of its natural oils that are crucial in keeping your hair healthy and shiny. For a natural conditioner, combine 1 tablespoon raw honey and 2 tablespoons coconut oil in a small bowl and mix well. Using your fingers, apply the mixture thoroughly to the bottom two-thirds of your hair while it is damp, starting at the ends and working up. For best results, let the mixture sit in your hair for 20 minutes then rinse with warm water.

MOISTURIZE CRACKED HEELS

Cracking on your heels can result from your skin becoming excessively thickened or too dried out. These cracks can range from minor to severe and can be irritating or painful. In a medium sized bowl, combine 1 cup raw, organic honey with 2 tablespoons milk and the juice of 1 whole orange. To make it easier to work with, try warming the honey slightly before mixing. Before applying the mixture, use a pumice stone to remove any excess calloused skin. Spread a generous amount of the mixture onto your

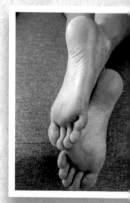

Soften calloused heels

heels and massage thoroughly to help your skin absorb the mixture. Let the mixture sit for 45 minutes, then rinse with warm water and dry thoroughly. Repeat this process twice daily. Alternately, you can apply this mixture to your heels and let it dry and leave it on overnight. You can also wrap it in gauze and leave it on overnight or while walking around. This mixture will keep up to 1 month in the refrigerator. Before each use, scoop 2 tablespoons of the mixture into a small bowl and place the bowl in hot water to make it easier to apply.

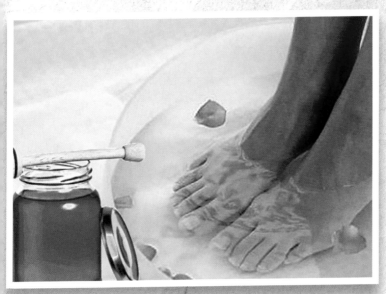

Honey foot spa

HONEY FACE MASK

Honey is a natural humectant, meaning it has the ability to hold onto water and can hydrate your face without leaving your skin feeling oily. Additionally, honey contains alpha hydroxy acids, which can encourage exfoliation and increases your skin's ability to absorb moisture and nutrients. By using honey as a face mask, you can relieve dryness and irritation in a natural way. Raw, organic honey is the best for a face mask as it has retained active enzymes that are beneficial for your skin. To use honey as a face mask, put 2 tablespoons raw honey in a small bowl. With went fingers, gently spread the honey onto clean, damp skin using circular motions. Let the honey sit for 30 minutes and then rinse your face well with warm water. Avoid using soap on your face after this process and follow up with your favorite moisturizer if desired.

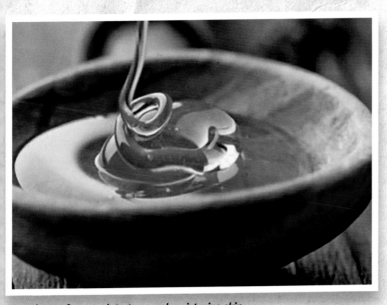

Use a honey face mask to tone and moisturize skin

BEAUTY/PERSONAL

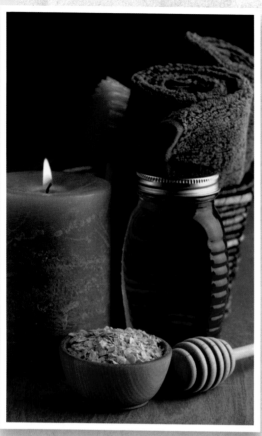

Honey and oatmeal

HONEY BATH

If you suffer from dry skin from sun exposure or winter months, try adding honey to your bath. For a moisturizing and relaxing soak, add 2 cups honey to your bath as the water is running. Soak for at least 15 minutes for maximum effect. For extra moisturization, follow up with a honey body scrub to remove any dead skin cells.

HAIR HIGHLIGHTER

Honey contains traces of hydrogen peroxide and can be used to lighten your hair gently. Honey contains the enzyme glucose oxidase which slowly releases hydrogen peroxide. Add 3 tablespoons raw, organic honey into 1 cup of warm water and stir well. Apply mixture evenly to your hair and let it sit for at least 30 minutes. You can even sleep with the mixture in your hair by wearing a shower cap. For best results, repeat the process weekly. For an extra lightening agent, try adding fresh lemon juice to the honey and water mixture. Before stirring in honey, combine one part fresh lemon juice with one part warm water. It is important to dilute the lemon juice to reduce the acidity and minimize any damage to your hair. Once you have stirred in the honey, apply to your hair evenly and let it sit for 30 minutes.

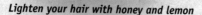

Lighten your hair with honey and lemon

FADE SCARS

Honey can lighten skin, and the anti-inflammatory and antibacterial elements can help to increase healing and decrease the appearance of scars. Make a mixture of one part raw, organic honey and one part

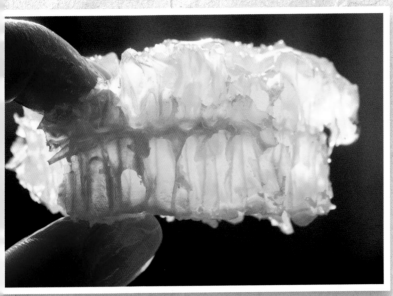

Use honey to minimize scarring

coconut oil. Using the tips of your fingers, apply the mixture to the affected area and massage into the skin in circular motions for up to two minutes. After two minutes, place a hot washcloth over the area and let it sit until cool. You can repeat this process daily to reduce the appearance of scars.

HEAL CRACKED CUTICLES

As honey is a natural moisturizer, it is an excellent remedy for cracked cuticles. Additionally, honey is loaded with enzymes and nutrients that will nourish and heal skin. For a balm that will quickly heal your cuticles combine 1 teaspoon honey, 1 teaspoon apple cider vinegar, and 1 teaspoon coconut oil in a small bowl. Using your fingers, rub

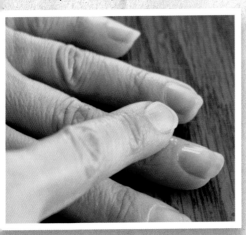

the mixture over your cuticles. Let the mixture sit for 10 minutes and then rinse with warm water. While honey would be moisturizing alone, the conditioning element of coconut oil and the acetic acid in apple cider vinegar will combine to be the most effective remedy.

Promote healthy cuticles

BEAUTY/PERSONAL

SOOTHE A SUNBURN

Honey can restore hydration to sun-damaged skin. Make a mixture of 1 part raw, organic honey and 2 parts pure aloe vera gel. Apply this mixture to sunburned skin for a cooling, moisturizing

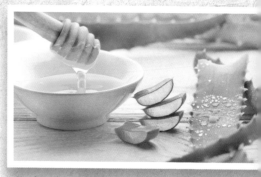

Heal sunburned skin with honey

effect. Both honey and aloe vera contain powerful anti-inflammatory properties to calm irritated skin and speed recovery.

LEMON RUB

Lemon and honey are both gentle and natural exfoliants. To give your face a deep clean, combine lemon and honey. Cut a lemon in half and remove any visible seeds. Apply 1 teaspoon raw, organic honey to the exposed surface of 1 lemon half. Rub the lemon half over your face, being careful to avoid eyes, adding honey to the lemon as necessary. Rub all over the face in circular motions and let it sit for 10 minutes before rinsing thoroughly with warm water. If you find that this method is too harsh for your skin, trying letting the lemon juice and honey sit for less time.

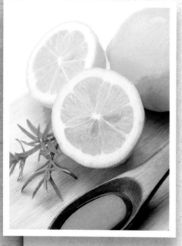

Exfoliate with honey

HAIR RINSE

Make a hair rinse with honey to give your hair extra shine and promote hair growth. In a small pitcher or jug, combine 2 teaspoons honey with 2 tablespoons apple cider vinegar and 1 cup warm water. Stir well to combine and set aside for use after your normal shampoo and conditioner routine. Pour the mixture evenly over your hair at most once a week to improve and regulate your hair's moisture.

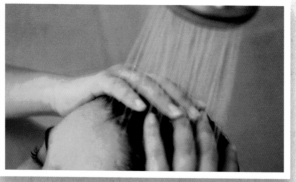

Make your hair shine

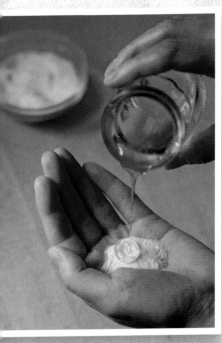

*ney and baking soda

BODY SCRUB

If you are looking for a natural, gentle body scrub, try honey. Make a mixture of two parts raw, organic honey with one part baking soda. Baking soda is a gentle mechanical exfoliant while honey is a natural chemical exfoliant. You can use this mixture from head to toe, starting at your feet and working up the body in gentle, circular motions to efficiently exfoliate your skin. Rinse with warm water when finished to reveal healthy and hydrated skin.

COMBAT ACNE

If you are suffering from a breakout, try using honey rather than a drying pimple cream. To combat a breakout, apply a very light layer of honey to the irritated area at night and wake to calmer skin. Simply apply a small amount of honey to a cotton bud and dab onto the skin. For an extra calming effect, try adding a drop of tea tree oil to the honey before applying.

Improve skin health

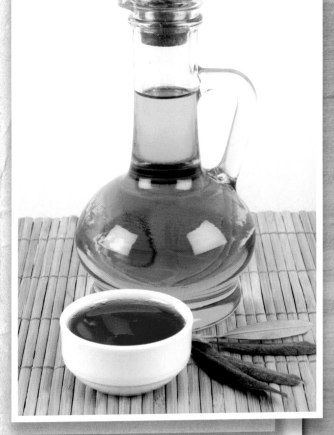

BEAUTY/PERSONAL

Beeswax Lip Balm

1 tablespoon beeswax, grated or pellets
1 tablespoon coconut oil
¼ teaspoon castor oil
1 tablespoon shea butter
(optional)
¼ teaspoon vanilla extract
(optional)
4 drops essential oil of choice
(optional)
Small containers or empty lip
balm tubes

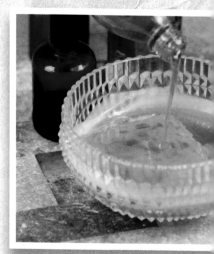

Make natural lip balm

In a small pan, melt coconut oil over low heat. Then add beeswax and shea butter and stir until all ingredients are melted and thoroughly combined. Add the castor oil, stir, and then remove from the heat. Let mixture cool until warm to the touch but not thick. Add optional vanilla and essential oils if desired and stir. While it is still liquid, pour into containers and let cool until solid.

Solid Beeswax Perfume

2 tablespoons beeswax
2 tablespoons coconut oil
Essential oils, 2 or 3 scents
Small containers, tins, or jars
To make your own solid perfume, you need to choose two or three essential oils that you like that work well together. For two scents, 30 drops of each will be sufficient, whereas for 3 oils, 20 drops each will be sufficient.

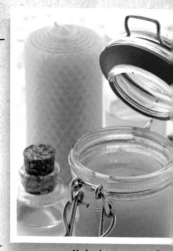

Make beeswax perfume

Create a double boiler using a glass jar or deep bowl and a saucepan. Place the jar or bowl in saucepan and fill the pan with water until it covers ⅔ of the jar. Put pan over medium heat and add beeswax and coconut oil to the jar. Stir often until liquid; once melted, carefully remove jar from heat and add essential oils. Stir well and immediately pour the mixture into any small tins or jars and let cool. Once the mixture has set, rub a small amount onto your neck and wrists and enjoy your new perfume.

Beeswax Lotion Bar

2 ounces beeswax grated or pellets
2 ounces coconut oil
2 ounces shea butter
10-20 drops lavender essential oil (optional)
½ ounce lavender buds (optional)
2 ounce silicone molds

In a small saucepan, combine beeswax, coconut oil, and shea butter. Over low heat, stir regularly until mixture becomes liquid, then immediately remove from the heat. Stir in essential oils and lavender buds, if desired, and pour into silicone molds. Set the molds aside until completely cool. Once cool, release the bars and store in a cool, dry place. To use, warm with your hands and rub over the skin as you would a traditional lotion.

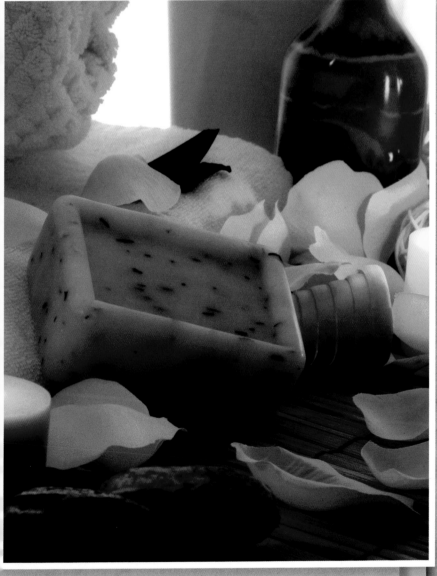

Make natural, healthy body lotion

HOME

Beeswax is the only naturally-occurring wax. Made exclusively by honey bees, beeswax is a byproduct of honey that bees create and use to build the comb structures inside their hives. Beeswax is well-known as an ingredient in natural lip balms and candles; its uses extend far beyond that. As beeswax has a low melting point of 140°F, it is very easy to work with for DIY projects. Beeswax is one of nature's most versatile substances.

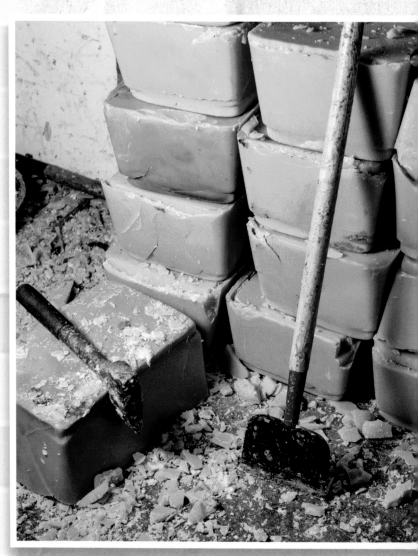

Solid beeswax

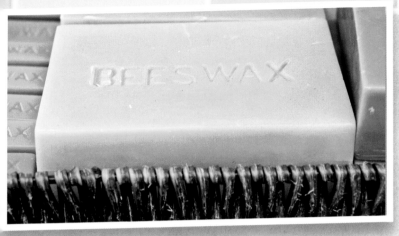

Beeswax soap

SMOOTHER WINDOWS

Take a solid block of beeswax and rub it onto any window tracks or drawer slides that stick to restore smooth movement. Beeswax is particularly good as a lubricant for oiling old furniture joints.

FURNITURE POLISH

To create a furniture polish, create a double boiler out of a short glass jar and pot of water. Combine 1 tablespoon grated or pellet beeswax with 3 tablespoons coconut oil in the jar. Boil the water in the pot until the wax and oil have melted, stirring often. Once melted, carefully remove the jar from the pot and let the mixture cool. Once the mixture has cooled and hardened, use a clean cloth or rag to rub into any wood furniture that needs polishing. Then, with a second clean cloth, buff the mixture into the furniture until any residue is removed.

COUNTER POLISH

To polish your granite countertops, use beeswax. Simply rub a small amount of warmed beeswax into the surface and allow it to dry. Repeat this process until your entire counter has been covered. Once dry, buff the counter to remove any excess beeswax. By applying beeswax as polish to granite countertops, you will keep the counters in good condition and help to prevent staining.

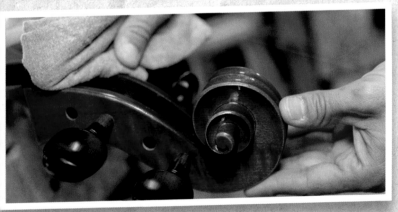

Polish and shine surfaces

HOME

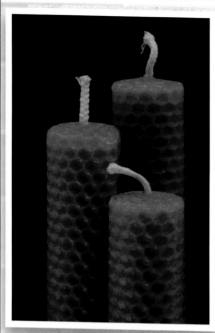

Make your own candles

DIY JAR CANDLES

Many scented candles can contain harmful ingredients, and regular scented candles are a huge source of indoor air pollution. Most scented candles are made of paraffin wax, which emits benzene and toluene when burned, which are both known carcinogens. Additionally, in the United States, candle wicks are meant to be made of cotton or paper; however, studies have found that almost 30 percent of scented candles contain some combination of heavy metals in the wicks. The artificial scents and dyes in many candles also release additional chemicals when burned.

By making your own beeswax candles, you are eliminating a harmful object from your home as well as purifying indoor air. Ready-made beeswax candles can be pricey to purchase, so making your own is an easy way to purify your home in a cost-effective way.

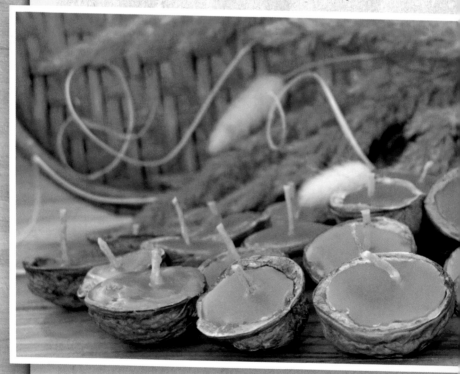

Beeswax Candles

This recipe makes 3 half-pint candles

1 pound pure filtered beeswax
½ cup coconut oil
3 8-ounce canning jars
60 ply cotton braided wick
1 metal pitcher or metal can
Large pot
Bamboo skewers
Essential oils (optional)

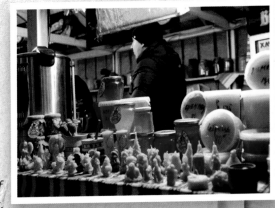

Beeswax candles

Place beeswax into the metal pitcher or can, then place pitcher into the large pot, and fill with enough water to cover two thirds of the pitcher. Over medium-high heat, bring water to a boil and maintain a gentle boil until beeswax has completely melted. To speed up this process, you may want to chop the beeswax into small pieces if you have a solid beeswax block.

While the beeswax is melting, cut the wick into 3 pieces, each 6 inches long. Once the beeswax is completely melted, remove pot from heat and add coconut oil to the pitcher. Stir gently using the bamboo skewer until coconut oil and beeswax are thoroughly combined. We recommend using a bamboo skewer as they are disposable and beeswax is very difficult to remove from surfaces.

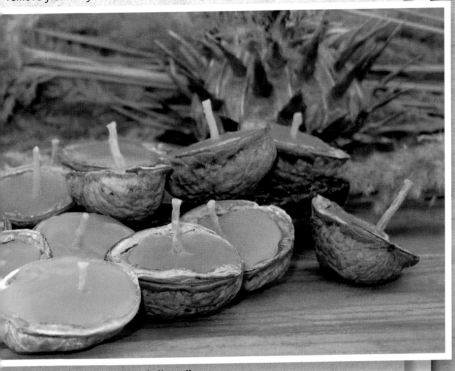

Homemade beeswax walnut shell candles

HOME

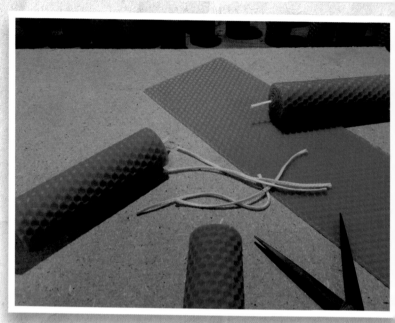

Materials for beeswax candles

One at a time, pour ½ inch of wax mixture into the bottom of each jar and return the pitcher to the hot water to keep the wax in a liquid state. Place a wick into the wax in the center of each jar, using another skewer to ensure the correct placement and to hold the wick until the wax is cool enough to hold the wick on its own. Once the wax is completely cool, approximately 5–10 minutes, take the top end of the wick and wrap it around a bamboo skewer until the wick is taut, then rest the skewer

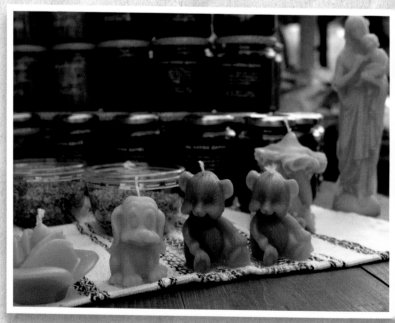

Environmentally friendly and pleasantly scented

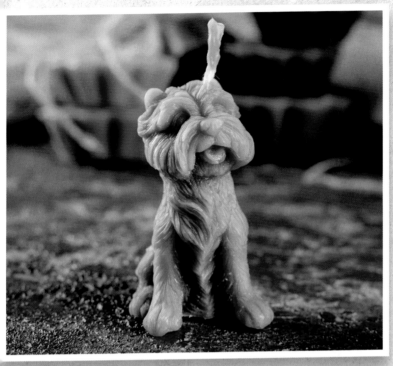

Long-lasting, eco-friendly candles

across the top of the jar. If necessary, use a small piece of tape to keep the wick attached to the skewer. Hold the skewer in place so that the top of the wick is centered in the mouth of the jar and carefully pour the remaining wax into the jar, leaving an inch of space at the top. Repeat this process for all 3 jars to create 3 candles.

Set the candles aside overnight so that they cool completely. Beeswax candles are known to crack occasionally, so to avoid this, set each jar in a bowl of warm water before setting it aside to slow the cooling process and lower the chance of cracking. Once completely cool, trim the wick to ½ inch. For best results, let the candle burn until the entire surface of the candle has melted the first time you use it to avoid the flame tunneling into the candle.

If you'd prefer to have your candles scented, you can add essential oils to your wax mixture. Beeswax does not hold scent as well as other waxes, but the addition of coconut oil will give the scent more staying power. Strong scents hold up best, such as peppermint and lemongrass. Experiment with essential oils to find what works best and is to your preference.

WARNING!
Beeswax is flammable, so be sure to keep an eye on it as it heats to avoid any accidents.

Once you have gotten comfortable with the process, you can make candles in any size jar. If you think you will make candles often, it is good to keep your metal can or pitcher as a dedicated beeswax container for future use.

Note: Some essential oils are toxic to pets and children, so be sure to check before making candles using certain essential oils.

HOME

DIY FOOD WRAP

While convenient, plastic wrap is terrible for the environment and completely unsustainable. It is a single-use petroleum product that is wasteful and can leach toxins into the food it comes into contact with. Fortunately, an alternative exists. Beeswax-coated cotton food wraps are reusable, safe, economical, functional, and eco-friendly. They are also very easy to make. If you are interested in lowering the amount of plastic in your kitchen, plastic food containers and bags can also be replaced by glass or stainless steel alternatives. Plastic wrap presents a greater challenge due to its convenience. To give beeswax-coated cotton wraps a try, just follow this recipe.

Beeswax-Coated Cotton Wraps

Beeswax, grated or pellets
100% cotton fabric
Cookie sheet
Wide paintbrush
Barbeque skewer
Twine
Clothespins or binder clips
Oven

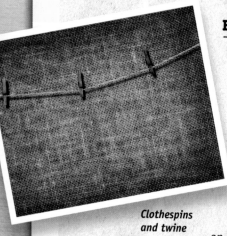

Clothespins and twine

Note: As beeswax is incredibly difficult to remove, it is best to use an old cookie sheet that will be dedicated to this purpose. You can try placing a sheet of parchment paper under the fabric but the beeswax may leech through. The same applies to the paintbrush you will use.

Preheat your oven to 185°F.

Use the twine to create a makeshift clothesline in your kitchen.

The best fabric to use is 100% cotton that has the thickness of a bed sheet with a very tight weave. Be sure to wash your fabric and allow to dry thoroughly before use. Cut your fabric to size, 12" x 12" and 8" x 8" squares are appropriate, and place the fabric on a cookie sheet. You will likely need to do one sheet at a time as you cannot overlap the fabric. Sprinkle your fabric evenly and lightly with some grated or pellet beeswax, approximately 1 ounce of beeswax per sheet. Once the oven has reached temperature, place the cookie sheet in the oven and watch carefully until the beeswax has just melted, about 5 minutes or less. As soon as the beeswax has melted, remove from oven and use your paintbrush to spread the beeswax to any areas that are not saturated.

Once the fabric is saturated, hang it on clothesline using clothespins or binder clips until dry. Once cooled, your beeswax-coated food wrap is ready for immediate use.

To use your new food wrap, place the wrap over a bowl or around food and hold with your hands. The heat from your hands will cause the wax wrap to mold and it will cool in the shape you held it in. You can also make smaller sheets to cover small containers such as jars. After use, clean your food wrap with cool water and mild soap. Using warm or hot water will cause the beeswax to melt and lose its function.

Note: If your wax hardens before it has been evenly spread, simply put it back in the oven and repeat the process until complete.

Note 2: If you have excess beeswax on the cookie sheet, you can place your next sheet on top and it will absorb the extra wax.

WARNING!
Be sure to place a sheet or dropcloth under your clothesline to catch any beeswax drips

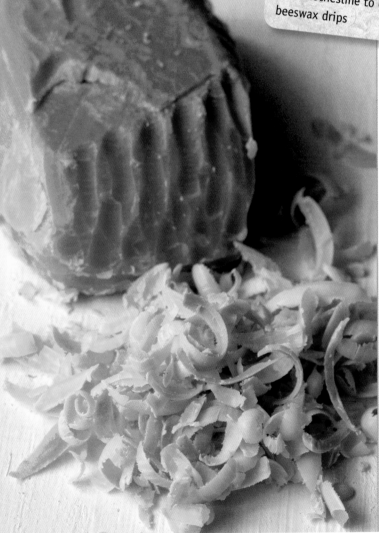

Grated beeswax

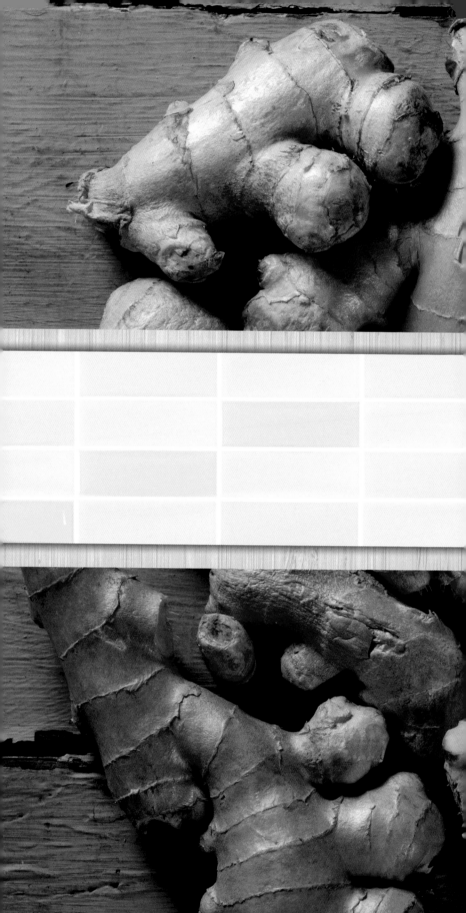

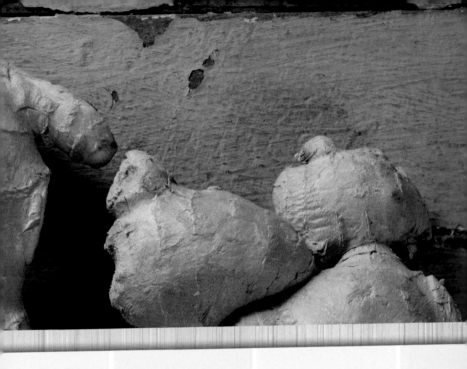

CHAPTER 7
GINGER

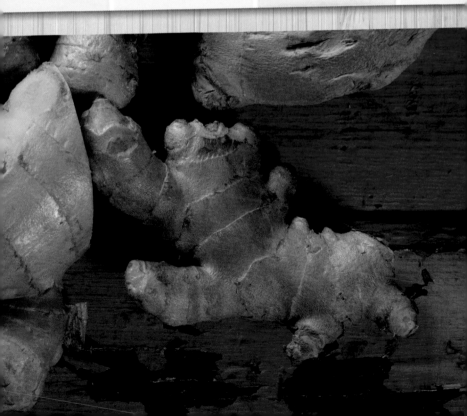

GINGER USES

Ginger is one of our oldest and most useful plants. For centuries, humans have used ginger in food, as a cosmetic, and even as homeopathic medicine. Ginger's natural properties allow it to help with just about anything from joint pain to digestion, making it a common solution for many people suffering from arthritis, nausea, and inflammation. It first originated in China before it was traded all over the world. and has since become a staple in just about every household and restaurant for its distinctive flavor and wide array of health benefits.

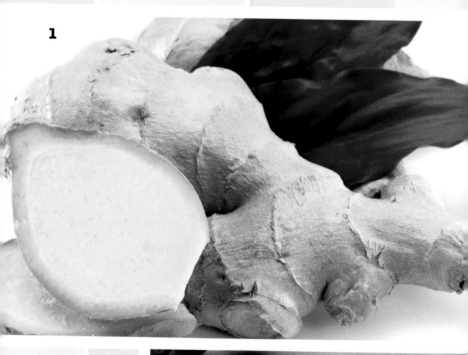

1

1 Sliced ginger
2 Ginger iced tea
3 Ginger and
   garlic
4 Ginger and
   lemon
5 Fresh ginger
6 Grated ginger

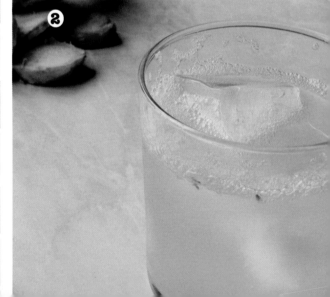

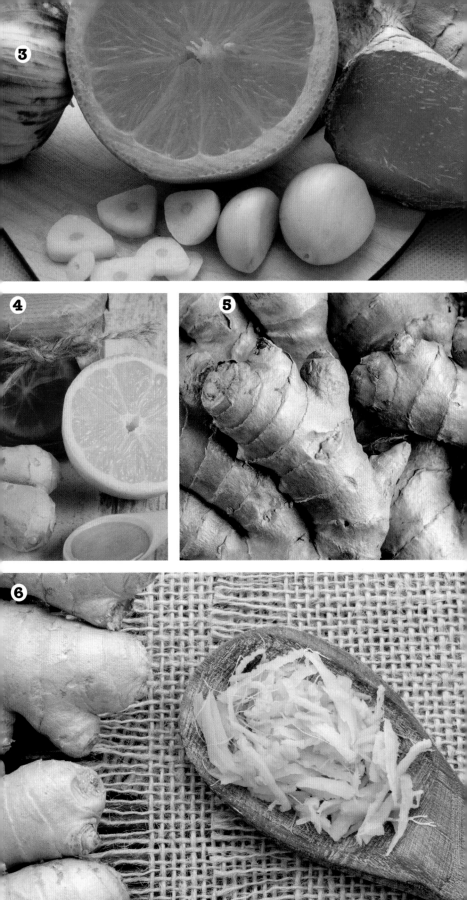

WELLNESS

Ginger isn't just used as a way to add a note of spice and heat to meals—it can also act as a surprisingly powerful medical supplement. It aids in everything from digestion to fighting cancer, and can also be used topically to fight infection and soothe the pain of minor cuts, scrapes, and bruises.

One of the best ways to use ginger is to simply add it to your diet as much as possible. Given the fact that ginger is known to boost your metabolism, raise your energy level, and diminish your chances of getting sick, a diet rich in ginger can improve your everyday health and state of mind more than you expect.

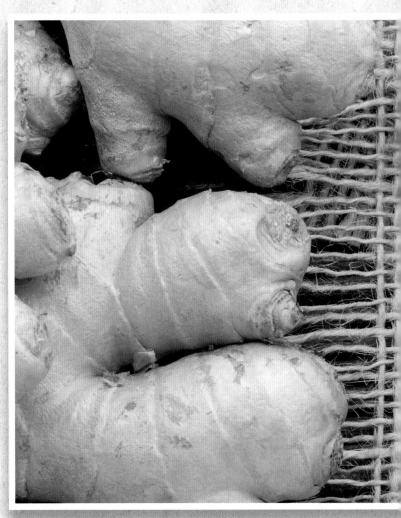

Raw ginger

AID DIGESTION

Eating raw ginger is a great way to relieve an upset stomach, no matter the cause. This is one of the easiest ways to help prevent vomiting, relieve stomach pain or nausea, and generally improve your digestive health.

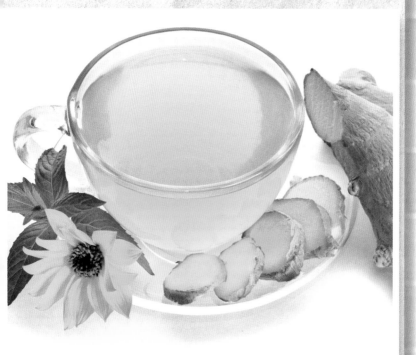

Ginger tea

EASE MOTION SICKNESS

If you struggle with motion sickness when riding in cars or on planes, chewing on some raw ginger—or on ginger candy, if you find the taste to be a little too strong—should help minimize your discomfort. At the very least, the sharp taste and smell of ginger will distract you from the movements of the vehicle, diminishing the mental part of the cause of motion sickness.

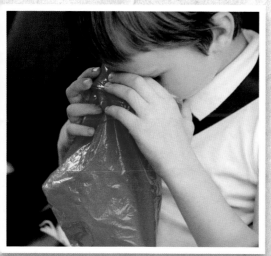

Treat motion sickness

WELLNESS

IMPROVE METABOLISM

Ginger can help you avoid getting an upset stomach in the first place by aiding in the production of digestive enzymes, breaking down proteins and allowing your body to absorb nutrients more easily. This will increase how efficiently you digest and metabolize your food, which will allow you to burn energy more efficiently and reduce the amount of fat that your body stores instead of burning. The better your stomach is at digesting food healthily and quickly, the less likely you are to experience stomach aches and discomfort.

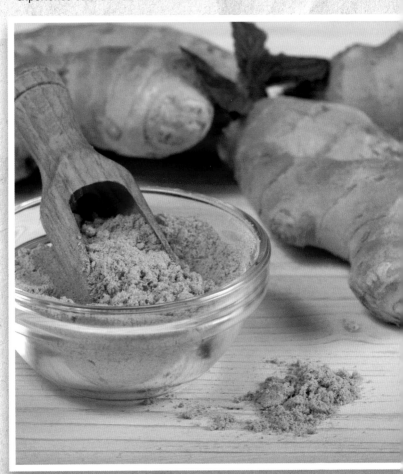

Speed up your metabolism

RELIEVE MORNING SICKNESS

As with motion sickness, you can relieve some of the discomfort of morning sickness during pregnancy by chewing a piece of raw ginger. Ginger is generally considered to be safe for pregnant women to eat, although you should always consult your doctor before consuming anything you think might be detrimental to your health.

LOSE WEIGHT

Ginger can be used as an appetite reducer by chewing a small piece before a meal; you should find yourself better prepared to eat smaller portions and less inclined to overeat. Portion control is a healthy tool for weight loss, as long as you make sure that you still get all the calories and nutrients you need with every meal.

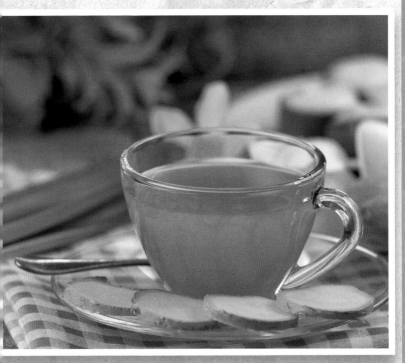

Improve digestion

REGULATE INTESTINAL FUNCTION

Ginger can help regulate the production of mucus in your body, which is vital to ensuring a healthy intestinal and digestive system. Grind 1 tablespoon fresh ginger into a powder and boil with water for a great-tasting and healthy tea that will help keep your digestive system working healthily.

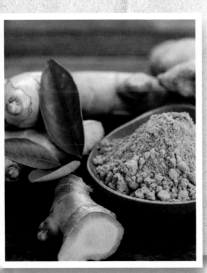

RELIEVE BLOATING AND GAS

To relieve bloating due to gas, you can crush or grind 1 tablespoon fresh ginger root and mix the powder into a glass of warm water to make a juice. Drinking this should help break down some of the gas in your stomach, relieving bloating and pain quickly and easily.

Ease bloating

WELLNESS

SOOTHE HEARTBURN

Ginger juice or tea can be also be used to treat heartburn, and to prevent it in the first place. Adding a fresh cup of ginger and lemon tea to your morning routine every day, or chewing ginger before every meal, can help keep your stomach acid settled, limiting the pain of heartburn and acid reflux. This is not a replacement for any medication you may have been prescribed, but it does serve as a quick way to minimize the discomfort of heartburn.

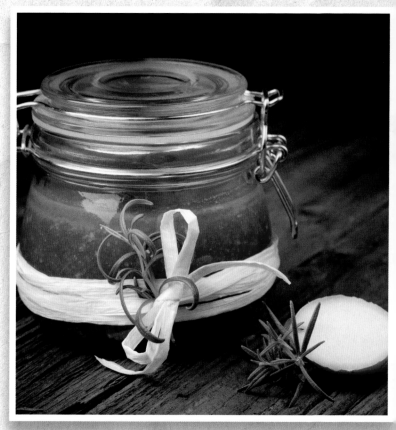

Soothe heartburn

PAIN RELIEF

Not only is ginger a natural digestive aid and antiemetic, it also has pain-relieving and anti-inflammatory properties that can be used to diminish muscle and joint pain, sore throats, and many other kinds of aches and pains.

WARNING!

While ginger can be a great pain reliever, it should not be used as a substitute for immediate medical attention. Always contact your doctor in case of injury or sickness before trying other options.

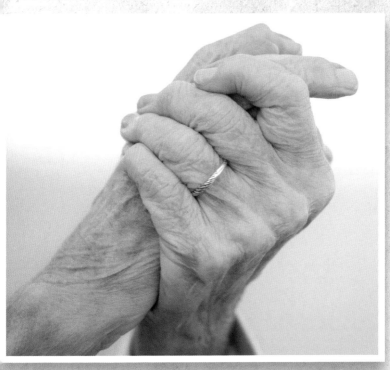

ase arthritis pain

RELIEVE ARTHRITIS PAIN

If you suffer from arthritis—or most other kinds of joint pain—you can use ginger to help lower swelling, relieve pain, and improve joint and muscle mobility. One method you might use is a ginger bath: add 1 tablespoon ginger essential oil to hot bath water, and soak in it for up to an hour. The combination of hot water, steam, and ginger should help soothe your joints and relax your mind and body, lowering stress and pain at the same time. For more immediate or location-specific results, you can also mix ½ tablespoon ground ginger and 1 tablespoon coconut oil into a smooth paste and massage it gently into your hands, knees, or any other afflicted area to help relieve pain and inflammation.

EASE SORE THROATS

Drinking ginger tea mixed with 1 teaspoon honey can soothe sore throats and help people get over colds more quickly. The ginger helps restore the health of mucous membranes that line your throat, relieve irritation, kill bacteria, and return you to good health in no time.

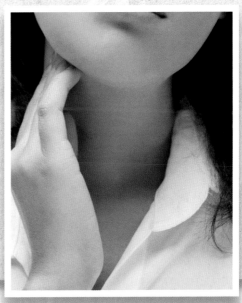

Calm sore throats

WELLNESS

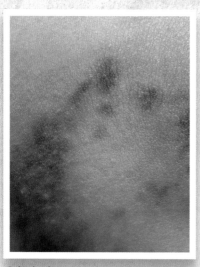

Calm bruises

CALM BRUISES, SWELLING, AND INFLAMMATION

Because ginger is naturally able to reduce pain, swelling, and inflammation, it's no surprise that ginger paste can be used to treat bruises and swelling. Simply grind fresh ginger down into a smooth paste and apply it liberally to the site of a bruise. You should feel a decline in pain and see the swelling start to go down before too long.

EASE MENSTRUAL PAIN

If you suffer from painful menstrual cramps, eating ginger is a proven way to help minimize your discomfort. Ginger tea, fresh raw ginger, or even a decent amount of ginger cooked into food will all help relieve pain and cramping. The soothing nature of ginger and lemon tea will also help you relax, distracting you from any lingering discomfort.

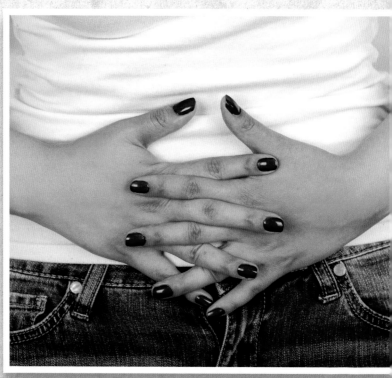

Ease menstrual cramps

QUIET HEADACHES

It has been suggested that, when crushed into a smooth paste—you may also want to mix it with coconut or almond oil—and applied to the forehead, ginger can even help cure headaches. While this may not be effective for a headache caused by dehydration, ginger will certainly help lower inflammation and relieve some topical pain.

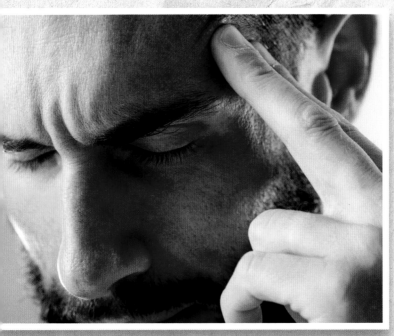

uiet headaches

SOOTHE BURNS

Ginger can also be used to soothe the pain of recent burns. Crush fresh, raw ginger into a paste and apply it liberally to the site of a minor burn to cool the irritated skin and promote healing.

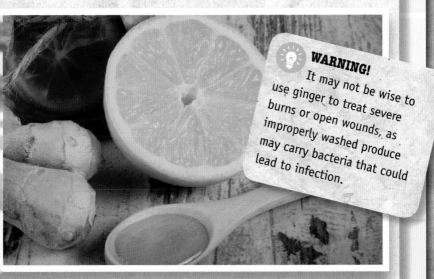

WARNING! It may not be wise to use ginger to treat severe burns or open wounds, as improperly washed produce may carry bacteria that could lead to infection.

oothe burns

WELLNESS

A diet that contains a regular amount of ginger can help fight off and prevent many illnesses. By fighting inflammation and infection, boosting your immune system, and even fighting cancer, ginger can be a vital part of keeping yourself in good shape for a long, healthy life.

HEART HEALTH

One of the most important ways to make sure you live a long, healthy life is to take good care of your heart. Heart disease and heart attacks can be avoided with a healthy diet, and careful management of your cholesterol. Ginger can help keep your heart healthy in both of these ways, as well as by providing a few other benefits. A diet rich in ginger has been shown to reduce cholesterol, decrease high blood pressure to safer levels, lower blood sugar, and promote healthy circulation and bloodflow. Keeping your heart in good condition will pave the way for a healthier life overall, reducing your risk of strokes, heart attacks, and disease.

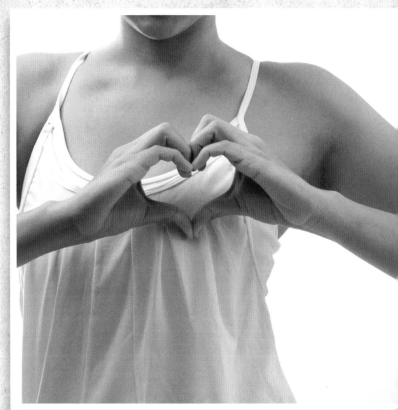

Heart disease and heart attacks can be avoided with a healthy diet

CONTROL ALLERGIES

Ginger is a natural antihistamine, so it can be a surprisingly efficient way to treat seasonal or pet-related allergies. Chew on a piece of raw ginger, or eat foods with lots of ginger in them. The spice of ginger should also help clear your sinuses a little, the way eating hot peppers does. You might also want to try drinking hot ginger tea—the steam may help relieve some of your congestion, as well as soothing any coughing or inflammation that comes with your allergies.

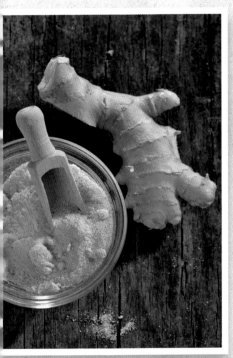

A natural antihistamine

Ginger can also help treat some of the symptoms of conditions such as asthma, although it should not be used as a replacement for prescribed medicine, especially in the case of an asthma attack.

SOOTHE ECZEMA

The rash that results from a bad case of eczema is essentially just another kind of inflammation, which ginger is adept at soothing. Taking regular doses of ginger—either in food, tablets, or in tea—provides effective and long-lasting relief from their symptoms.

BOOST IMMUNE SYSTEM

Ginger has quite a few antiseptic qualities, which—combined with keeping injuries from becoming inflamed—can help keep infections at bay when applied to minor cuts, scrapes and burns. It also helps keep your immune system strong

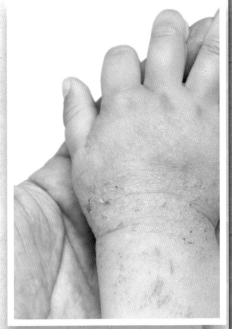

Regular doses of ginger provide effective relief from the symptoms of eczema

when eaten regularly, which allows your body to put in more work when preventing and recovering from infections.

WELLNESS

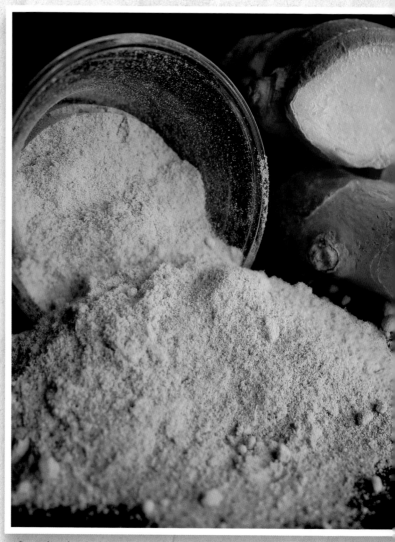

Ground and raw ginger

PROMOTE LIVER HEALTH

Unsurprisingly, ginger can help keep just about every part of your body healthy. The liver, for example, benefits greatly from regular ginger supplements. The liver and kidneys help filter toxins out of your bloodstream and then flush them out of your system. While they should be working just fine on your own, ginger helps that process along. This can be especially helpful for anyone suffering from an increase in liver toxicity, or just as a way to help you get your personal health back where you want it to be. It has also been suggested that ginger can help the liver control and minimize any harmful side effects of prescribed medicine, which—especially when treating serious diseases—can be quite hard on the liver.

AVOID KIDNEY STONES

Kidney stones are uncomfortable, painful, and can even result in hospitalization or surgery if your body can't deal with or avoid them on its own. While a healthy diet should normally prevent the kind of calcium buildup that causes kidney stones in the first place, regularly drinking strong ginger tea can help your body break down kidney stones and avoid ever allowing them to form. By keeping your kidneys healthy in the same way that it protects your liver, ginger can make them run as efficiently as possible. You will also be more hydrated if you regularly drink ginger tea, which is vital to proper kidney function and the avoidance of kidney stone development.

FIGHT ALZHEIMER'S AND MEMORY LOSS

One of the key factors that accelerates the progress of Alzheimer's disease is chronic swelling or inflammation of the brain. Inflammation of the brain for extended periods of time slowly damages your brain's ability to send and process information, resulting in the gradual breakdown of your neural pathways. Because ginger is a strong anti-inflammatory, making it a regular part of your diet may help prevent or fight the development of conditions such as Alzheimer's disease.

PREVENT CANCER

Tumors are formed when cells in the body become mutated, and do not go through their normal life cycle and instead continue to grow and multiply. Ginger contains a compound called 6-gingerol, which could help prevent tumor growth by helping these cells die instead of rapidly multiplying. Ginger is thought to be especially useful in preventing the growth of tumors associated with cancers of the pancreas, prostate, and ovaries.

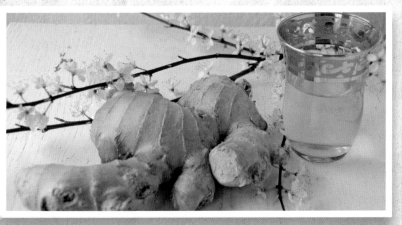

Help reduce your risk of cancer

BEAUTY/PERSONAL

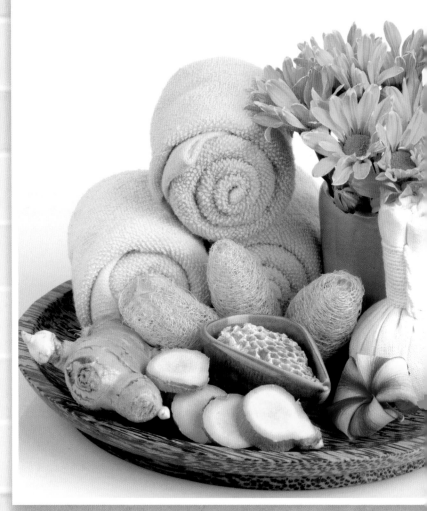

Use ginger to soften and rejuvinate your skin

Because of its ability to reduce inflammation, promote skin and cell health, and fight bacteria and fungus of just about any kind, ginger makes a great addition to your skin and hair-care routine. Simply eating a regular diet of ginger should keep you healthy and energized every day, but you can always go the extra mile by making facial scrubs, skin toners, and even hair growth tonic to get as many of ginger's benefits as possible.

Because ginger naturally reduces pain and inflammation, ginger baths, scrubs, and foot soaks are also a great way to reduce your stress levels at the end of a long day or when you feel like treating yourself.

Minimizing stress is one of the most important ways you can take care of your health and appearance, and will also simply make you feel better in the long run.

REDUCE WRINKLES

Ingesting ½ tablespoon crushed ginger with 1 tablespoon honey, or drinking ginger tea daily, helps to reduce wrinkles. This works primarily because ginger has a high antioxidant content, which reduces the speed at which skin ages. Ginger also helps your body prevent elastin from breaking down, which would otherwise cause wrinkles.

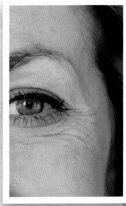

Smooth wrinkes

TREAT ACNE

Ginger contains a plethora of chemicals that help reduce pain and skin inflammation caused by acne. In addition, ginger kills bacteria that causes acne and promotes proper circulation, both of which contribute to healthier skin. Chewing a small piece of ginger root or drinking ginger tea twice a day will give the body the antioxidants needed to maintain healthy skin.

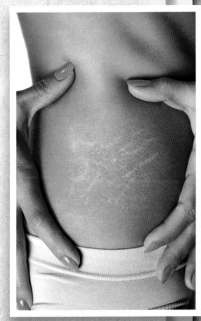

REDUCE STRETCH MARKS

An effective home remedy for stretch marks is to make a body mask of ½ tablespoon dried ginger root, 1 tablespoon shea butter, and 1 tablespoon coconut oil. These ingredients nourish your skin, help fight toxins and free radicals that cause stretch marks, help the skin heal faster, and prevent stretch marks from reoccurring.

Reduce stretch marks

BEAUTY/PERSONAL

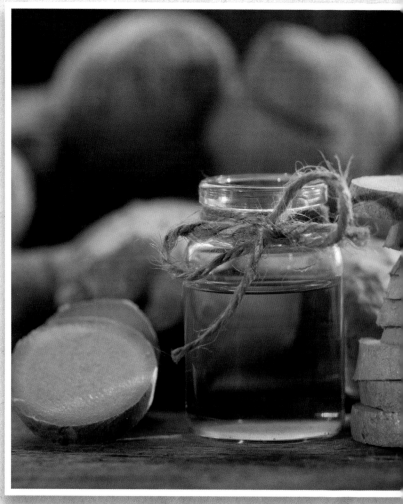

Chopped ginger and ginger oil

REDUCE CELLULITE

For those struggling to minimize cellulite, ginger has been known to revitalize skin, making it smoother and healthier. Although the exact cause of cellulite is unknown, it believed to be caused by fat cells protruding into the outer layers of skin. A lemon-ginger body scrub can rejuvenate the skin and reduce cellulite.

Lemon-Ginger Body Scrub

1 tablespoon ginger root
1 tablespoon sugar
1 tablespoon olive oil
1 tablespoon lemon juice

Mix all ingredients into a smooth paste and apply to face and body once a week.

TONE SKIN

Ginger can be just as useful at improving the quality of your skin even if you aren't affected by acne, age spots, or stretch marks. The antioxidant properties of ginger are known for softening the skin and evening out the skin's complexion, and reducing inflammation should keep away any puffiness, redness, or blotchiness in your face. Use a face mask of 1 tablespoon ginger juice, 1 tablespoon rosewater, and ½ tablespoon honey every morning—along with a cup of strong ginger tea—to keep skin looking healthy and rejuvenated.

FADE SCARS

Ginger can be used to treat scars, especially acne scars, due to its natural anti-inflammatory characteristics. It contains antioxidants such as vitamin C, which is highly effective as speeding up healing time of scars. Ginger can be used as a component of a face mask in addition to honey and water, or small pieces of fresh ginger can be placed directly onto scars as spot treatment. This should be done no more than once a week, as skin is very sensitive to ginger.

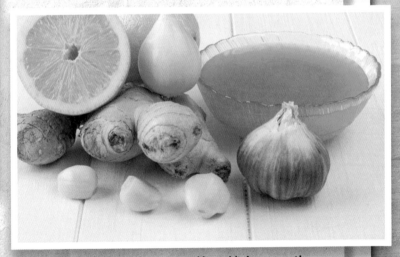

Ginger makes a great addition to your skin and hair-care routine

EXFOLIATE HAIR FOLLICLES

In order to maintain healthy hair, it's necessary to exfoliate dead skin cells and get rid of clogged hair follicles. Ginger is rich in vitamins and minerals which can be used for exfoliation. It promotes oxygen flow to the roots and its moisturizing and antifungal properties also prevent dandruff. To use it as an exfoliant, combine 1 tablespoon each crushed ginger, honey, and baking soda and massage the paste gently into your scalp. Rinse clean with warm water and follow up with your preferred shampoo or conditioner. Repeat this once a week, or twice a week for a more thorough cleanse, but no more frequently than that in order to avoid doing more harm to your scalp than good.

BEAUTY/PERSONAL

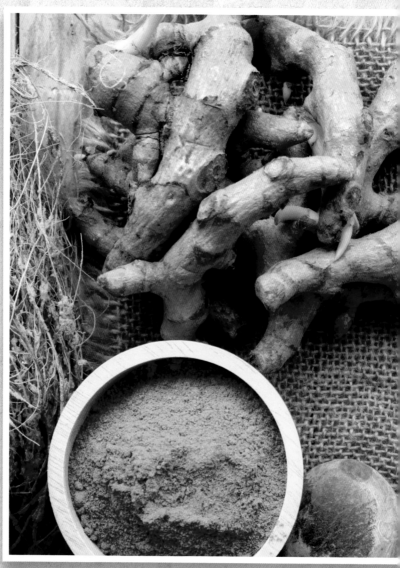

Powdered ginger

PREVENT SPLIT ENDS

Ginger's naturally high number of antioxidants are essential for repairing damaged hair. For split ends, consider a mixture made of chopped or ground ginger root, aloe vera, and olive or coconut oil. These ingredients will condition and detangle your hair, in addition to combatting split ends and returning your hair to its proper shine. Mix ½ tablespoon ginger, 1 tablespoon aloe vera, and ½ tablespoon coconut oil into a smooth paste and use it as you would shampoo. Rinse your hair thoroughly and follow up with a gentle conditioner. Try this once a week for best results, but avoid repeating it daily to keep your hair from becoming too oily.

PROMOTE HEALTHY HAIR

Ginger is an organic remedy that can condition the hair to improve both its look and feel. The oils in ginger contain antioxidants which revitalize hair and protect against damage. Add 1 teaspoon crushed ginger to your conditioner to maintain a healthy head of hair. Ginger contains many vitamins and minerals that stimulate hair follicles, strengthen hair strands, and promote hair growth. In addition, it keeps hair healthy and moisturized to prevent future hair loss. A hair mask can be created by combining 1 tablespoon ginger root and 2 tablespoons almond oil and massaging the mixture onto the scalp.

LESSEN DANDRUFF

Ginger naturally contains antiseptic properties which kills the fungi that cause dandruff. Combining ½ tablespoon each ginger juice and lemon juice with 1 tablespoon yogurt and applying to the roots of the hair will combat dandruff and keep the scalp moisturized. This removes dead skin cells and prevents the dandruff from reoccurring.

STRESS RELIEF

For stress relief, soak your feet in a mixture of 2 tablespoons mustard powder, 2 teaspoons fresh grated ginger, 1 cup mint leaves, and enough warm water to cover your feet and ankles up to your lower shins. After a few minutes, your aching feet will hurt less, and you will feel a noticeable drop in stress and anxiety.

Tip: Hot water will make the mustard less effective, so use warm or lukewarm water instead.

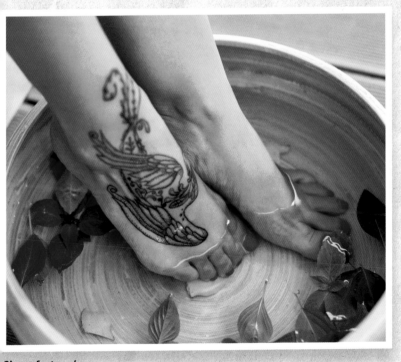

Ginger foot soak

BEAUTY/PERSONAL

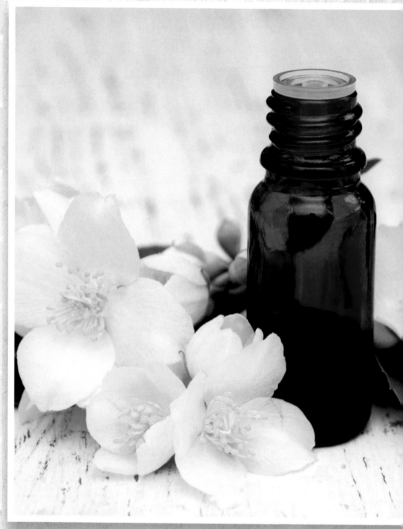

Ginger essential oil

GINGER AND ROSE MASSAGE OIL

Infuse any oil of your choice (olive oil and coconut oil are great, inexpensive options) with ginger and rose to make a romantic, warming massage oil. In a glass container, mix 1 cup oil, 10 small organic dried rosebuds, and 2 teaspoons fresh or dried ginger.

Tip: Add a few drops of rosemary essential oil for preservation purposes if you plan on keeping it for a while.

Tip 2: To speed up the infusion, place all ingredients in a saucepan and simmer over low heat for about 45 minutes. Let cool to room temperature and pour into a glass container.

CIRCULATION AND RELAXATION BATH

You can use ginger to make your own bath salts, which will improve your circulation, soothe your tired or aching muscles and joints, and help you relax after a long day at work. In a jar, mix ¼ cup coarse sea salt or Epsom salt with 3 teaspoons ginger and ½ teaspoon of cinnamon. Add the whole mixture to a hot bath, and soak for up to an hour for optimal relaxation and stress relief.

Tip: Feel free to add a few drops of the essential oil of your choice! You might want to try lemon, orange, or grapefruit, as the citrus pairs especially well with ginger.

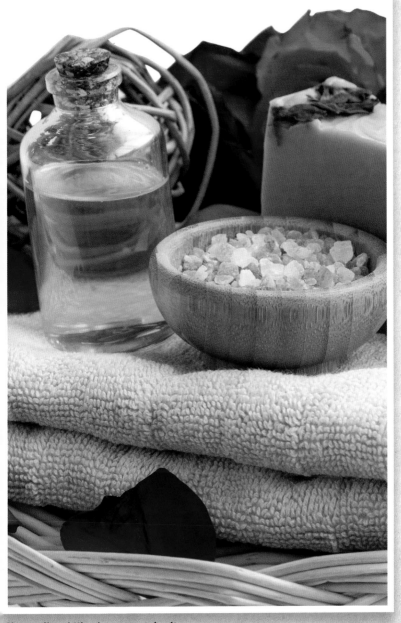

Ginger oil and Himalayan crystal salt

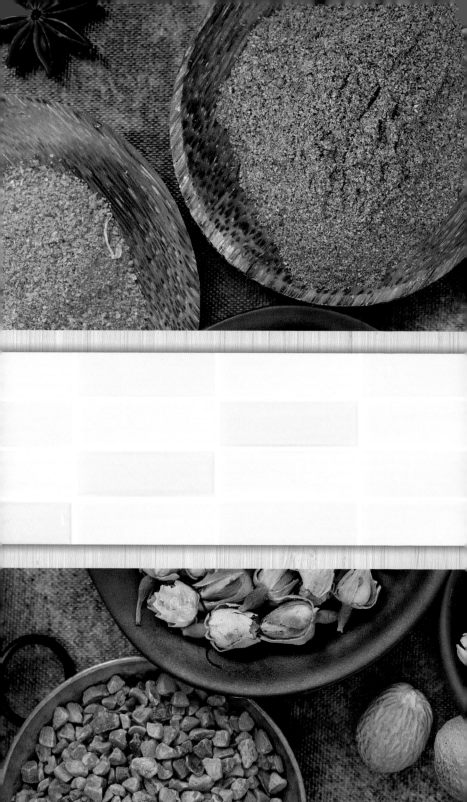
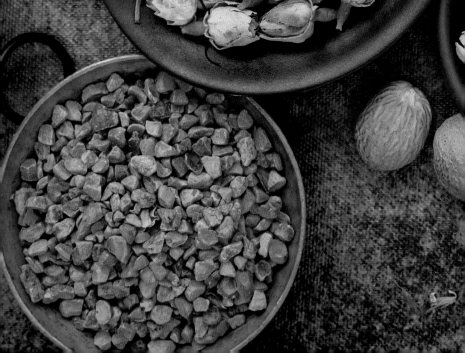

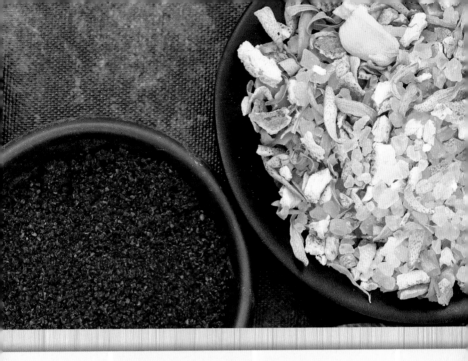

CHAPTER 8
OTHER NATURAL INGREDIENTS

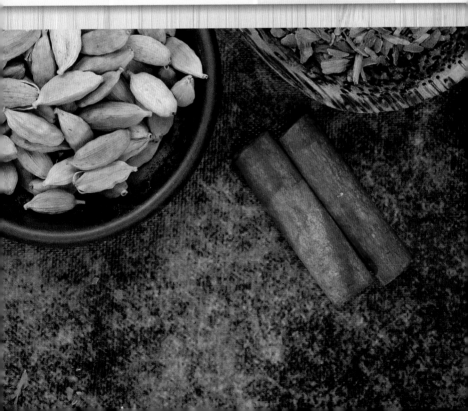

OTHER NATURAL INGREDIENTS USES

There are countless uses for some of the everyday items you can find around your house or in any standard grocery store. From scouring pots and pans with lemon juice to fighting sickness with ginger, there are hidden uses and benefits to just about everything. Here's a quick overview of some other popular items that have surprising wellness, beauty, and home uses. As always, it pays to do your research, and to figure out which of these uses works best for you. With any luck, you might just come across a few cheap, healthy, effective ways to improve your quality of life.

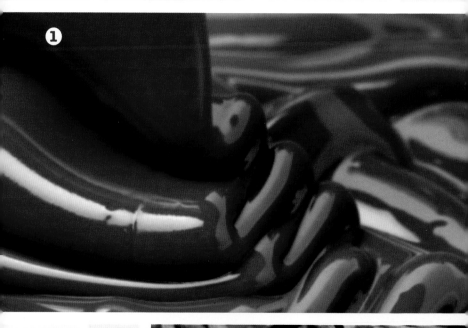

1 Dark chocolate
2 Cloves
3 Turmeric
4 Black pepper
5 Borax
6 Garlic

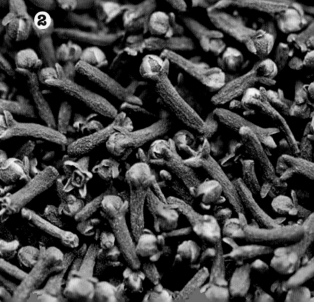

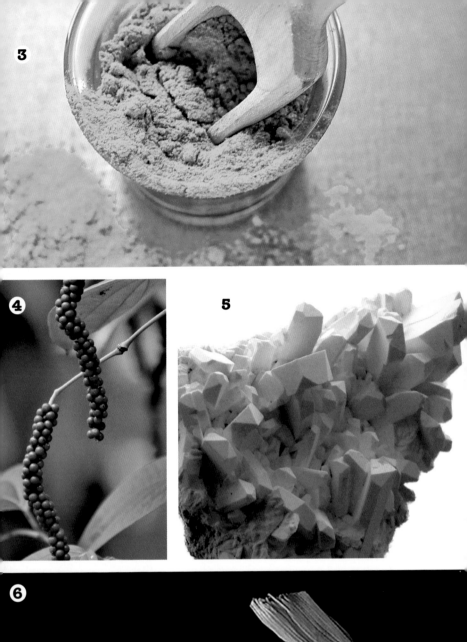

3

4

5

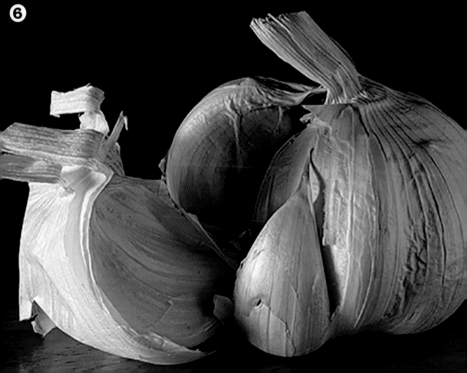

6

DARK CHOCOLATE WELLNESS

Chocolate has been one of our most valuable and widely appreciated commodities for the last few centuries or so. We've praised it for its flavor as a dessert in cakes, cookies, and just about every other kind of dessert you can think of—but chocolate has a number of powerful wellness benefits that you can take advantage of to improve your health, happiness, and overall sense of well-being.

One of dark chocolate's most valuable benefits is its high antioxidant count. Antioxidants help rid your body of free radicals, which—when allowed to go unchecked—can cause cell mutations, prematurely

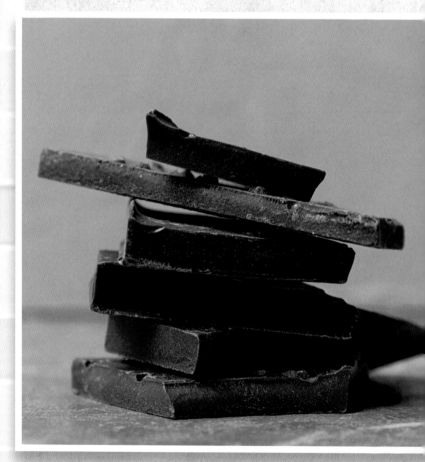

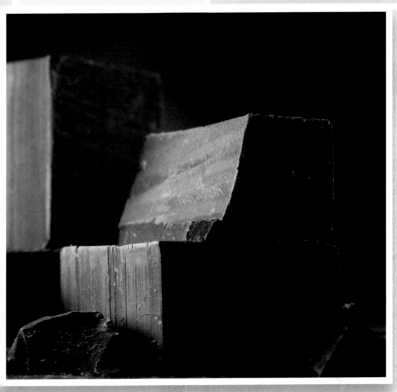

Dark chocolate chunks

accelerate the aging process and lead to wrinkles and skin discoloration, and increase your risk of dozens of other unpleasant conditions. Dark chocolate can also strongly affect your mood, reducing stress and increasing your energy levels, as well as reducing hair loss and even helping you lose weight. You can have access to all of these health benefits, while at the same time satisfying your sweet cravings with something that's actually good for you.

Chocolate was first cultivated in the Americas, with evidence of its use in society dating all the way back to the Olmecs, the first known major civilization to be established in Mexico. This traces the usage of chocolate as a food, medicine, and drink back as early as 1200 BC, some 3,000 years ago. Since then, it became a staple of most Mesoamerican cultures, and was so highly valued at some points that it was granted religious significance and even used as currency. It was first spread to Europe and, later, the rest of the world, when Spanish conquistadores arrived in the Americas in the 16th century. Within a hundred years or so, it had become a key part of European trade and culture, expanding into a massive industry for the next several centuries.

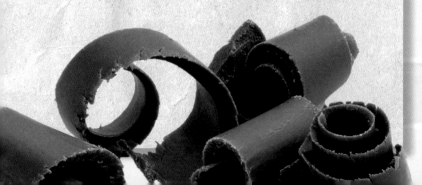

DARK CHOCOLATE WELLNESS

MOOD BOOSTER

Managing your stress levels is one of the best ways to stay healthy, and it can be one of the most difficult things to do when you're juggling work, family, and your own health. Dark chocolate is well-known for its ability to improve your mood in both an acute and long-term sense.

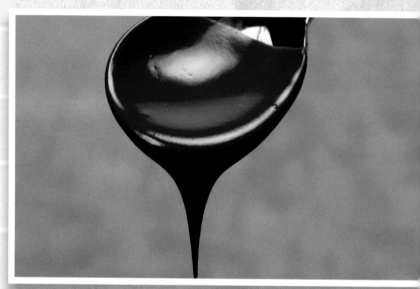

Improve your mood

Dark chocolate helps your brain produce endorphins more efficiently, which means it literally helps you feel happier, more relaxed, and less stressed. A little dark chocolate every day can help stave off stress, anxiety, and depression. The fact that it simply tastes good also helps, as sometimes all you need after a long day is a small treat.

APPETITE SUPPRESSANT

When you're hungry, it can be easy to give into your cravings for quick, unhealthy snacks to tide you over

Appetite suppressant

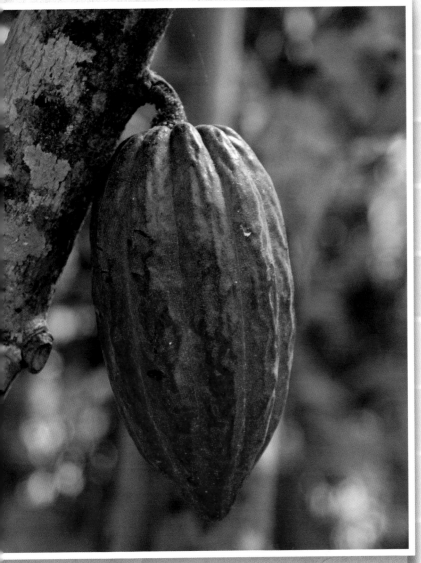

Cocoa bean pod

during the long hours between meals. It's good to keep your metabolism working consistently, but snacking unhealthily counteracts any benefits you might receive from that practice. Dark chocolate—even as little as a single square—is a great way to satisfy your cravings for sweet foods, while also helping you avoid overeating when your next meal arrives.

HEALTHY ALTERNATIVE TO CAFFEINE

Another quick, healthy way to incorporate dark chocolate into your daily routine is to use it as an alternative to your morning coffee, energy drink, or any other source of caffeine. As chocolate contains a chemical known as theobromine—similar in many ways to caffeine—it can give you a nice boost of energy, without being as hard on your stomach and teeth as coffee or as sugary and unhealthy as energy drinks. Theobromine also has less of a crash than caffeine-based products, so you won't find yourself falling asleep in the middle of the day when

DARK CHOCOLATE WELLNESS

it starts to wear off, and you won't be jittery or anxious while it's working.

Tip: If you're not quite ready to kick your coffee habit, try melting some dark chocolate into your coffee. It will improve the flavor while also giving you the benefits of dark chocolate, keeping you from having to go for a second cup anytime soon.

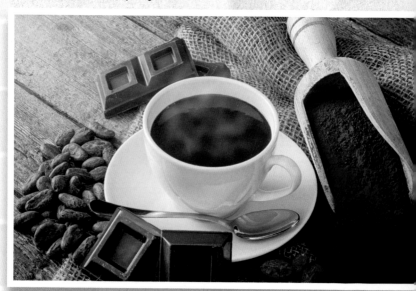

Add dark chocolate to your morning coffee

HIGH IN NUTRIENTS

Despite its reputation as a dessert, dark chocolate is actually surprisingly good for you. For one, it contains a large quantity of flavonols, as well as several chemicals that promote good circulation and blood flow, helping lower blood pressure and increase heart health. It also carries a fair number of the vitamins, minerals, and nutrients that humans need to stay happy and healthy. A good rule of thumb to keep in mind is that the darker the chocolate—meaning the higher the percentage of cocoa to other ingredients—the better it is for you.

Improve your health

PROMOTES A HEALTHY PREGNANCY

Pregnancy can be a difficult and complicated process to navigate, and it's hard to keep track of all the ways to avoid complications and ensure the health of your child. Dark chocolate—aside from satisfying one of the most commonly experienced pregnancy cravings—is useful for its ability to prevent a condition known as preeclampsia, which raises a pregnant woman's blood pressure to harmful levels, sometimes resulting in early labor or even death. Theobromine, the same chemical that can help boost your energy, helps lower blood pressure and improve circulation, lowering your chances of experiencing this condition. Chocolate is also high in antioxidants which help strengthen your immune system, another aspect of your health that is vital to ensuring a healthy pregnancy.

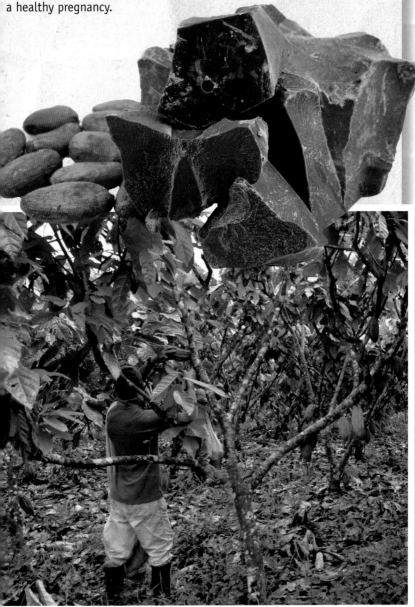

Harvesting cocoa in Ecuador

DARK CHOCOLATE WELLNESS

EYESIGHT

The high flavonoid count in very dark chocolate also helps improve bloodflow between your eyes and brain. This can improve your eyesight, most notably by allowing your brain to process the images your eyes receive more quickly.

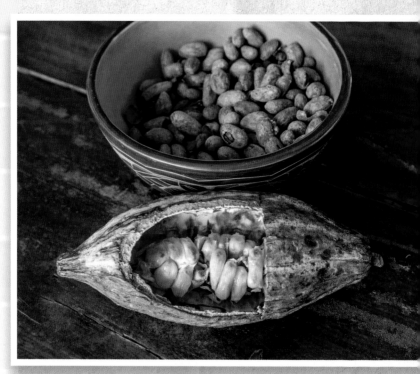

Opened fruit and seeds of the cacao tree

PROTECT SKIN FROM UV DAMAGE

Interestingly enough, one of the best ways to protect your skin from sun damage is to eat dark chocolate regularly. The best results will come from chocolate that is as close as you can get to pure cocoa, as the process of refining and sweetening chocolate can rob it of some of its flavonoids, reducing its antioxidant properties. Very dark chocolate can actually help protect your skin from ultraviolet light, minimizing burns and discomfort.

WARNING!

Always wear sun protection when going outside on a sunny day. This will help protect your skin or a regular basis, but shouldn't be used as a replacement for sunblock, especially if you have sensitive skin.

STROKE PROTECTION

Once again, the high flavonoid content of dark chocolate comes into play. In this case, dark chocolate has been linked to the reduction of the risk of having a stroke. It's not yet certain whether this decrease is a direct result of regularly eating dark chocolate, as opposed to an indirect effect of one of dark chocolate's many other health benefits, but either way, this is one of a surprising number of health benefits offered by dark chocolate.

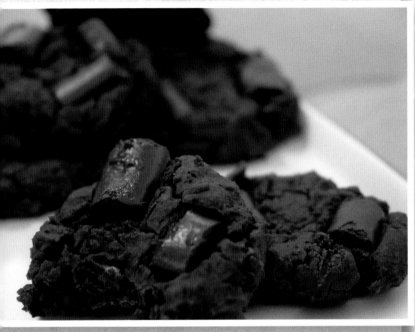

Avoid strokes

COGNITIVE FUNCTION AND MEMORY

One of the most well-known health benefits of dark chocolate is its impact on your brain's ability to store and process information. By increasing blood flow to your brain, dark chocolate helps you form new neural pathways quickly, helping you learn and memorize information more efficiently and increasing the speed at which your brain is capable of accessing those memories. As your neurons function more and more efficiently, you will find yourself more readily able to adapt to and understand new situations and concepts. The long-term implication is that you may be more likely to avoid memory deterioration later in life, as the breakdown of neural pathways is one of the primary causes of memory loss.

Improve memory

DARK CHOCOLATE WELLNESS

HEART DISEASE

Because dark chocolate is excellent at lowering your blood pressure, it takes no great leap of imagination to see that it can also help keep your heart healthy, preventing heart disease by avoiding buildup in your arteries and keeping your blood pressure low. The antioxidants present in dark chocolate can also help you avoid heart disease.

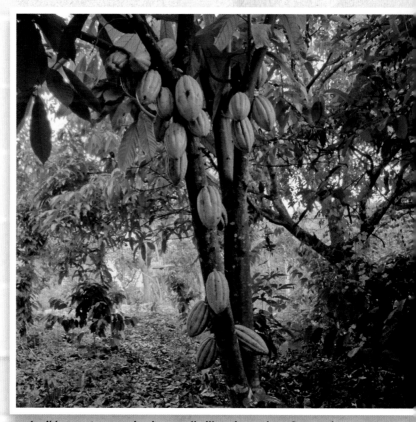

A wild cacao tree growing in a small village in northern Guatemala

BLOOD SUGAR

Oddly enough, chocolate—despite the fact that it usually contains a decent amount of sugar—can help you keep your blood sugar in check. The reason this works, assuming you're eating dark, good quality chocolate, is that dark chocolate can actually increase your body's sensitivity to insulin. This means that, despite the sugar present in the chocolate itself, the overall effect is that your body will be better equipped to break down all the sugar you eat, keeping your blood sugar from getting too high.

CHOLESTEROL

Dark chocolate with especially high percentages of cocoa has been shown to reduce cholesterol levels. The more cocoa present in the chocolate, the higher the levels of flavonoids, which contribute directly to increasing heart health, lowering cholesterol, and improving circulation.

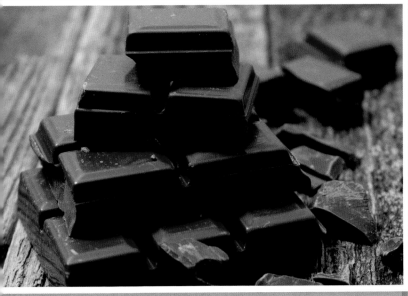

Lower cholesterol

ANEMIA

Anemia—a condition that results from a dangerously low red blood cell count, resulting in fatigue and malnutrition—can be treated with a supplementary intake of iron and vitamin C. Iron is the primary factor here, as your body needs it in order to produce enough red blood cells, while vitamin C makes your body better at absorbing iron from the food you eat. Chocolate is rich with iron, as well as many other trace elements, and can naturally help you improve your red blood cell count. Anemia can also damage your circulation, which is another area where dark chocolate has seen some positive results.

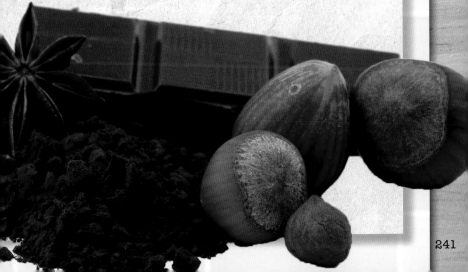

DARK CHOCOLATE
BEAUTY/PERSONAL

PROMOTE SKIN HEALTH

Regularly eating very dark chocolate can be a great way to keep your skin in good shape. Cocoa is nutrient rich and naturally helps you absorb other nutrients more easily, as well as protecting you from UV radiation—all of which help your skin stay healthy and smooth,

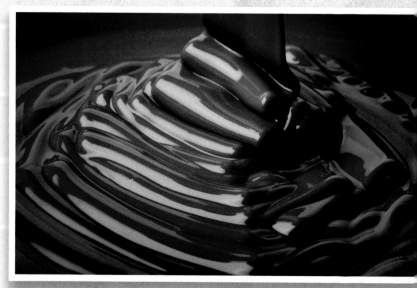

Get healthier skin

avoiding the development of wrinkles or discoloration. Dark chocolate also helps your skin stay moisturized rather than drying out, largely due to improved circulation and cell regeneration, as well as decreasing stress that might otherwise lead to acne breakouts or dark circles under your eyes. You can even apply it to your skin directly by incorporating raw cocoa powder into an exfoliating facial or body scrub. Mix together 2 bars melted dark chocolate, ¾ cup milk, 1 teaspoon sea salt, and 3 tablespoons brown sugar to make your own dark chocolate face scrub.

PREVENT HAIR LOSS

One of the main factors that contributes to hair loss is poor circulation. A lack of enough blood flow to the scalp can lead to hair falling out and not growing quickly enough, resulting in embarrassing bald patches. As chocolate improves blood circulation throughout your whole body, adding it to your diet is a great start to improve your hair's growth. On top of that, chocolate is rich in copper, zinc, and iron; all of which help produce cells faster and grow hair more efficiently.

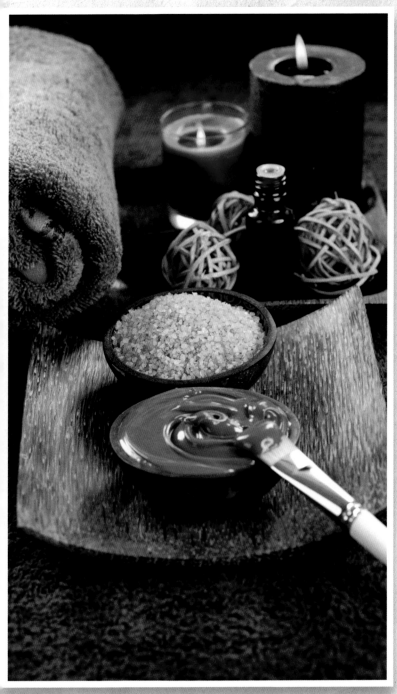

Keep hair healthy

HAIR HEALTH

You can improve the shine, volume, and texture of your hair by wrapping it with a mask of very dark chocolate—as close to raw as you can get—along with coconut oil, honey, or even yogurt. If you leave this mixture on your hair for an hour or two and then rinse thoroughly, you should immediately notice that your hair is shinier and more voluminous than before.

DARK CHOCOLATE BEAUTY/PERSONAL

DARK CHOCOLATE FACIAL

When used correctly, dark chocolate can be as great for your skin as it is for the rest of your body. The antioxidants in dark chocolate help slow the aging process, keeping your skin looking healthy and youthful, and incorporating a few other rejuvenating ingredients can give you a perfect face mask to use whenever you feel like treating yourself a little.

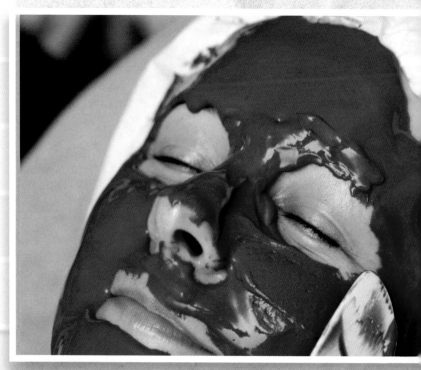

Dark chocolate face mask

Dark Chocolate Face Mask

All you need is 2 teaspoons pure cocoa powder, 1 teaspoon honey, and 1 teaspoon yogurt. Mix all your ingredients into a smooth, chocolate-colored paste, and then apply the mask onto your face in an even layer. Sit back and let the mask work for up to 30 minutes, then rinse your face with cool or warm water and a dry with a soft, dry cloth.

DARK CHOCOLATE BODY MASK

Just as you can use dark chocolate to brighten your complexion, you can apply a chocolate mask to your whole body for even more effective, relaxing results, or even make an exfoliating scrub with dark chocolate.

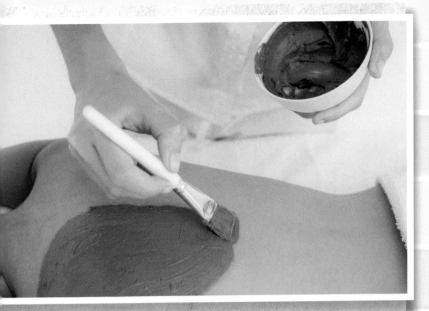

Dark chocolate body mask

Dark Chocolate Body Mask

Mix 4 tablespoons raw honey, 4 tablespoons pure cocoa powder, 1 tablespoon plain greek yogurt, and 2 teaspoons thoroughly ground oatmeal into a smooth paste. (You can make more or less depending on how much you think you'll need, or make a big batch and save some for later.) Use this mask as you would any other body mask, then rinse clean with warm water.

Exfoliating Dark Chocolate Scrub

Combine ½ cup brown sugar with either ½ cup cocoa powder or 1 bar of melted (but not hot) very dark chocolate and ¼ cup coconut oil. Mix everything into a smooth paste and gently scrub into any dry skin for a few minutes, then rinse clean with warm water.

DARK CHOCOLATE MASSAGE OIL

If you're looking for a Valentine's Day gift for your partner, making your own dark chocolate massage oil might be a good start. It's great for your skin, and a massage is a great way to reduce stress and improve mental health. Try melting down a bar of very dark chocolate along with two tablespoons coconut oil and one tablespoon cocoa butter in a saucepan, stirring constantly. Once it's cooled down but still soft, you might also want to include a few drops of an essential oil of your choice for added effect. Make sure to wait until the result is a smooth paste that is no longer hot to the touch before using it as a massage oil. Feel free to experiment with different ingredients to get your massage oil to the right consistency—adding more cocoa butter might make the result a little thicker, while almond or olive oil will do the opposite.

TURMERIC WELLNESS

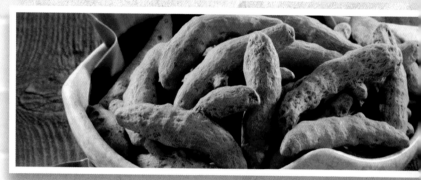

Raw turmeric root

Like its close relative, ginger, turmeric is capable of providing a vast array of health and wellness benefits when used correctly. Most of these benefits come from a chemical called curcumin. Also present in high quantities in ginger, curcumin is responsible for turmeric's signature bright yellow color and many of the significant health-improving qualities it can supply.

Turmeric is credited as the key ingredient in dozens of homeopathic treatments, and has been an important medicinal root for centuries. You can use it topically to reduce inflammation and relieve the pain caused by conditions like arthritis, or make it a regular part of your diet to improve your heart health and circulation, boost your immune system, and even speed up your metabolism a little.

Turmeric's powerful anti-inflammatory, antioxidant, and antibacterial properties make it an essential component of any natural medicine cabinet, and it can go a long way all on its own towards keeping you healthy all on its own.

Known also by its botanical name *Curcuma Longa*, turmeric is native to India. While in the modern day it has become widespread enough to be present on shelves in supermarkets and natural medicine stores all over

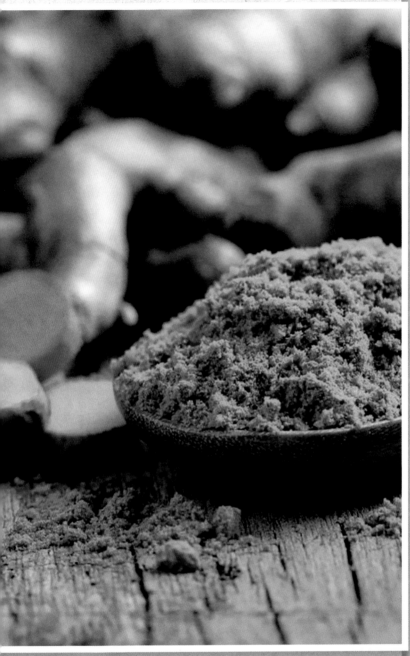

Ground turmeric

the world, it was first used in India as a spice and medicine for hundreds of years. It has also been used to make religious garments and wedding clothes, traded as a commodity, and has served as a brightly-colored and highly valuable dye for centuries.

Turmeric powder

TURMERIC WELLNESS

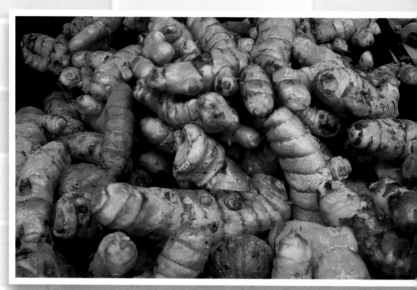

Fight free radicals

ANTIOXIDANTS

Turmeric is high in antioxidants, which allow it to rid your body of excess free radicals before they can do much harm. Free radicals occur when a molecule of oxygen separates into two individual atoms with unpaired electrons, which then roam your body in search of another atom to pair with, wreaking havoc along the way. These free radicals can be the catalyst for dozens of different diseases, many of which can be debilitating or even fatal. Antioxidants like those found in turmeric perform the important task of eradicating free radicals and other waste products on a cellular level, keeping you and your cells in a healthy balance. This is a vital aspect of human biology, allowing us to stave off heart conditions, limit our risk of diseases and mutations such as cancer, and slow visible signs of aging.

ANTI-INFLAMMATORY

Like its cousin ginger, turmeric is a surprisingly strong anti-inflammatory agent. It is extremely effective when used to reduce joint pain caused by inflammation and swelling, such as the joint inflammation that comes with arthritis. In some cases, sufferers of chronic joint pain have reported seeing better results with turmeric than with over-the-counter painkillers, although these results may vary from person to person. If you find that standard anti-inflammatory medicine isn't working for you, you might want to try turmeric and see if you get better results. This can apply to just about any condition that causes pain through inflammation, including anything from a bruise to an infected tooth.

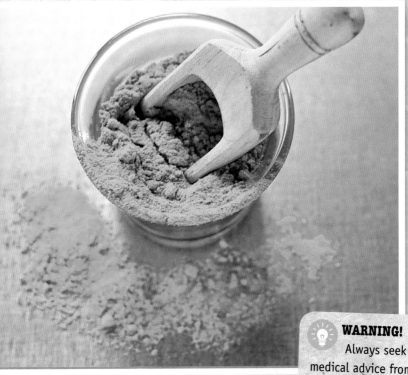

Reduce inflammation

PREVENT BLOOD CLOTS

This next usage for turmeric has the potential to be something of a double-edged sword. Turmeric is capable of thinning your blood almost as strongly as a prescribed anticoagulant, which can help prevent blood clots and keep your arteries healthy and your circulation in good condition. However, you should take great care to avoid using turmeric in combination with other medicine, as it may magnify the effects of other blood thinners or anticoagulants. Too much blood thinner in your system can result in nosebleeds, and even small cuts may bleed heavily and heal more slowly than usual.

WARNING!

Always seek out medical advice from a doctor before turning to homeopathic treatments, especially if you are concerned you may react negatively to the treatment in question.

HEART HEALTH

Keeping your heart in good condition should be one of your first priorities when thinking about your health. Many of our most fatal diseases are linked to poor heart health, blood pressure, and cholesterol—these can all be avoided with the right diet and lifestyle.

TURMERIC WELLNESS

Because turmeric is capable of preventing blood clots and clearing arteries of potential blockages, it can be a great help in your efforts to keep your heart healthy and your circulation unimpeded. By preventing blockages and keeping your heart going strong, you put yourself at less of a risk for heart attacks, heart disease, strokes, and high cholesterol.

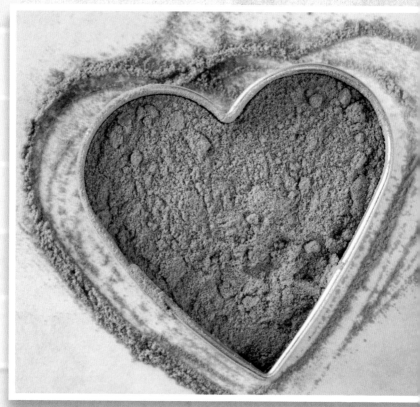

Promote heart health

LIVER HEALTH

Because of its natural ability to improve circulation and flush toxins from your bloodstream, turmeric is a perfect way to aid your liver in detoxifying your body. By providing more blood to your liver, turmeric will help your liver process and clean more blood more quickly, as well as aiding in the production of several enzymes that contribute to the repair, efficiency, and upkeep of your liver and kidneys.

CANCER PREVENTION

If you need any one reason to add a healthy dose of turmeric to your diet, the fact that it can be instrumental in preventing cancer should convince you. Curcumin, a chemical that is present in large quantities in both turmeric and ginger, has been shown to help fight cancer cells and inhibit their production. This is a vital aspect of cancer prevention, as minimizing the reproduction speed of cancer cells will slow the growth of malignant tumors, as well as helping your immune system by killing cancer cells throughout your body.

DIABETES

It seems as though diabetes is becoming more and more common with each year. One way you can avoid diabetes is by incorporating turmeric into your diet. Turmeric makes your body more receptive to insulin, helping regulate your blood sugar content and it from reaching

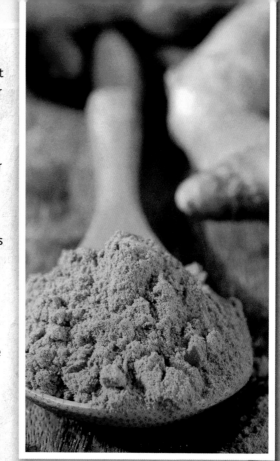

Reduce risk of cancer

especially unhealthy levels. This works best with a healthy amount of diet and exercise, as your body still needs to do some of the work, but turmeric should make preventing diabetes in the first place much easier. The increased receptiveness to insulin may also help those currently suffering from diabetes, but you should definitely check with your doctor first to see if it will interact with other medications you may be taking.

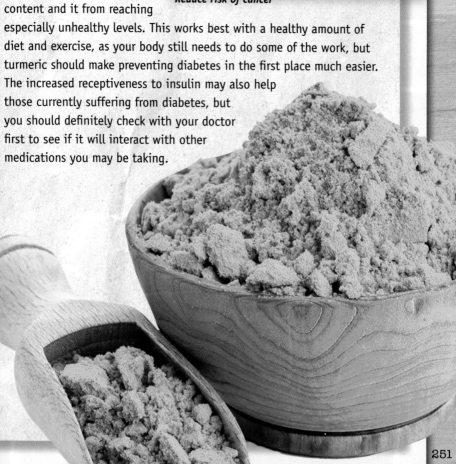

TURMERIC WELLNESS

IBS

Irritable bowel syndrome, or IBS, is an uncomfortable and stressful condition that can have a pretty severe impact on your daily life. While IBS is largely related to issues with your diet and stress levels, turmeric can help treat the symptoms of pain and discomfort by reducing inflammation in your stomach.

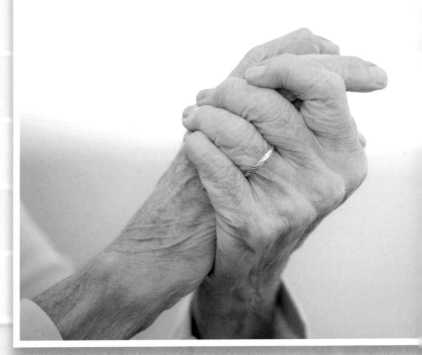

Ease joint pain

ARTHRITIS AND JOINT PAIN

Like ginger, turmeric has powerful anti-inflammatory properties. While this can help with a great number of conditions, its effects are most noticeable when used to treat joint pain caused by conditions like arthritis. Those suffering from arthritis experience severe inflammation in their joints, which can restrict mobility and cause a great deal of pain. Turmeric can help limit that inflammation, contributing directly to a reduction in pain and stiffness. This isn't a complete cure, however, just a way to manage the symptoms present, so you should not use this as a replacement for other medicines that may be intended to treat the cause.

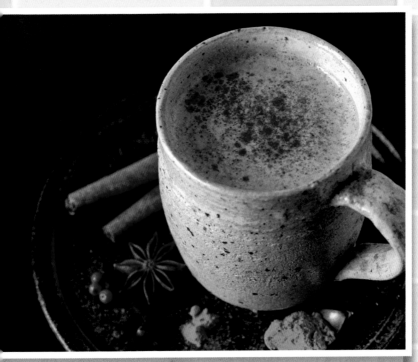

Sleep better at night

SLEEP AID

Not getting enough sleep is one of the easiest ways to cause long-lasting harm to your body. Sleep deprivation weakens your immune system, slows your reactions and brainpower, and can lead to weight gain, breakouts, depression, and anxiety. For those struggling with insomnia or having difficulty sleeping, turmeric might be able to help. In a glass of warm milk—soy or almond milk are also options, depending on your preference—combine 1 teaspoon ground turmeric, 1 teaspoon honey, and ½ teaspoon cardamom. This should help you relax and get to sleep better, instead of tossing and turning for hours.

BRAIN FUNCTION

For centuries, we have used turmeric to improve brain functions such as long term memory retention and concentration. Today, these benefits are still recognized. Tumeric increases blood flow to the brain and reduces inflammation, both of which can keep your neural pathways healthy and improve your cognitive function. Eating turmeric daily will help you focus on important tasks and aid memory retention.

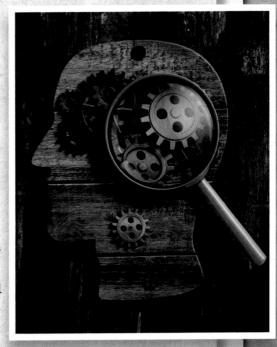

Improve cognitive function

TURMERIC WELLNESS

DEPRESSION

Depression is a difficult condition to manage, and it can be hard to find the right medication and treatment that works for you. Many people who suffer from depression and anxiety have found that ground turmeric can help boost their mood and give them more energy, reducing the often debilitating symptoms of these conditions. If you can't find a medication that works for you—or if you don't feel comfortable using antidepressants—this may be a good route to explore, with the bonus of having little to no side effects.

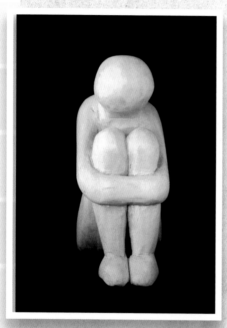

Fight depression

ALZHEIMER'S

Alzheimer's disease is a severe, damaging condition that slowly degrades your ability to form and access memories, and is often eventually fatal. One of the main factors that contributes to Alzheimer's is a buildup of plaque in the brain, which can cause neural pathways to deteriorate and inhibit cognitive function. Turmeric helps limit the formation of this kind of plaque, allowing your brain to continue working as normal, essentially helping prevent the early stages of Alzheimer's. Alzheimer's also causes inflammation in the brain, which turmeric's anti-inflammatory properties can help minimize.

UPSET STOMACH

Turmeric can be use to settle an upset stomach by improving the production of stomach acid that is necessary for healthy digestion. If the acidity of your

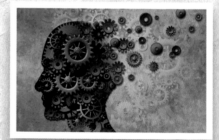

Reduce risk of Alzheimer's

stomach is out of balance, eating raw or ground turmeric can help return your digestive system to normal. Some have also found that turmeric can help reduce the discomfort of bloating, heartburn, and gas.

JAUNDICE

Jaundice is an unpleasant condition, but can be treated relatively quickly and easily with a healthy diet, lots of sunlight, and a doctor's visit if your symptoms are especially bad. One way to speed the healing process along is to put 1–2 teaspoons ground turmeric in your food or drink with each meal. Combined with a dedication to a healthy diet, this should help clear up your symptoms quickly and easily.

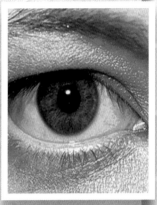

Help treat jaundice

INTESTINAL WORMS

This is an especially unpleasant and potentially dangerous condition, and you should certainly see a doctor if you think you might be experiencing it. However, turmeric is surprisingly capable at ridding your digestive system of intestinal worms—try drinking a glass of warm water with a few teaspoons of dissolved turmeric several times a day to help flush out any harmful bacteria lingering in your digestive system. This should not be used as a replacement for conventional medicine, however, unless you are advised to do so by a medical professional.

BURNS

To help reduce the pain and swelling that comes hand in hand with a burn, try mixing turmeric with cooling aloe vera and applying the paste to the surface of your wound. Turmeric has natural antiseptic and anti-inflammatory properties, which will help keep minor to moderate burns from becoming infected and minimizing some of your pain. Re-apply this mixture three times every day, and you should see results quickly. The aloe vera should help reduce your chances of scarring by moisturizing your skin and promoting cell reproduction, as well as cooling the burn and reducing pain and redness.

ECZEMA

If you suffer from eczema, you've probably already tried just about everything possible to find relief from the uncomfortable itchy, dry skin that it causes. Because turmeric is capable of killing harmful bacteria and reducing inflammation, it has been shown to provide noticeable relief from the symptoms of eczema when applied topically. Try mixing turmeric with coconut oil or aloe vera and spreading it on any areas affected by the rash, or simply rinse your skin with a mixture of ground turmeric dissolved in warm water.

Relieve eczema

TURMERIC BEAUTY/PERSONAL

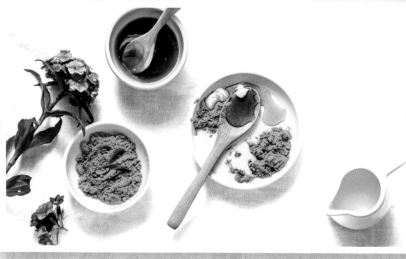

Turmeric, milk, and honey

ACNE

Turmeric is a great way to treat acne. It kills bacteria, reduces redness and inflammation—a staple of all acne breakouts from mild to severe—and can help clean pores that contribute to breakouts. Use ground turmeric in your next facial scrub to help cleanse your skin of these unsightly and painful spots, followed by a thorough rinse with cool water and then a soft, dry cloth. Repeat this every morning and before you go to bed at night for the best results, and you should see your acne begin to fade within a few days.

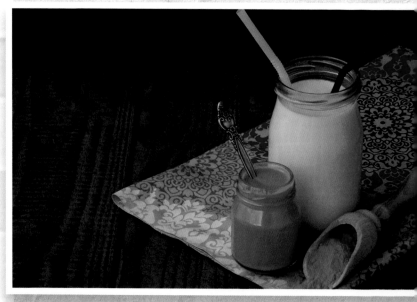

Fight acne

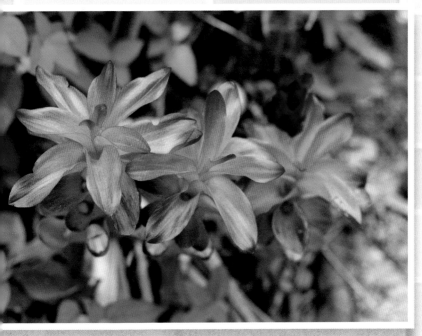

Turmeric flower

SKIN CARE

Taking care of your skin is a good way to minimize stress and improve your self esteem. Healthy, clear skin will make you feel better about the way you look, and will reduce your risks of break-outs and redness. Turmeric is great for treating dry or oily skin, helping you achieve a healthy balance between the two. A facial scrub consisting of ground turmeric, sea salt, and coconut oil will help clear out your pores and wash away excess oil on your skin, while also exfoliating and moisturizing dry or flaky skin. Washing your face with turmeric every morning and night should keep your skin healthy and moisturized.

WEIGHT LOSS

Losing weight is hard, especially if you have dietary, monetary, or medical restrictions that make it difficult to get enough exercise or maintain a healthy diet. Turmeric can help give your metabolism and digestive system a boost, allowing your body to burn excess fat faster and get the most out of any exercise you can get. The faster your metabolism is, the faster your body burns stored energy—this will help you lose weight and use up excess calories. For best results, combine a regular intake of turmeric with daily cardio-based exercise, and limit the amount of sugar-heavy foods you consume.

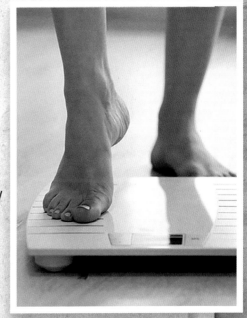

Promote weight loss

CLOVES

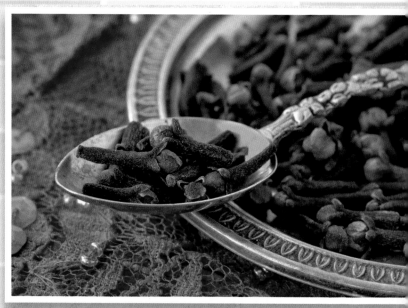

Cloves

Cloves are a staple spice in most kitchen cabinets, and are immediately recognizable for their unique shape and rich aromatic properties. They are native to the Maluku Islands in Indonesia, and were not cultivated anywhere else in the world until the 1700s. For centuries, the islands where cloves were grown put measures in place to limit their sale and exportation to other countries, but clove seeds were eventually spread outside of Indonesia, to be grown and sold elsewhere, and are now commonly bought and sold all over the world.

Since the earliest record of their existence, cloves have been put to a vast number of both culinary and medicinal uses. Cloves can be used to make spicy food richer and more flavorful, freshen breath, create a fragrance pomander in a fresh orange, and even serve as homeopathic medicine. As they have many anti-inflammatory properties and antioxidants, cloves can be useful either when eaten or when applied topically to aching joints and muscles.

Freshen breath and flavor food

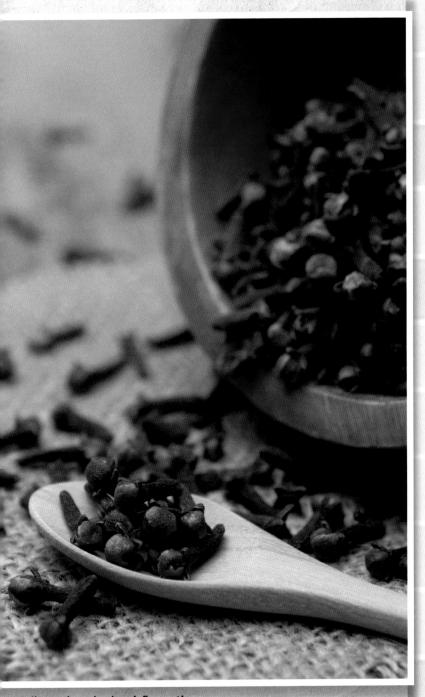

Relieve pain and reduce inflammation

Clove-based essential oils are also very useful, as they provide a concentrated way to access the active chemicals that make cloves so useful in the first place. The active chemical compound found in cloves is called eugenol. Eugenol gives cloves their pain-killing and anti-inflammatory qualities, and can often be found in extremely high concentrations when extracted as clove essential oil. Eugenol is also often used in perfume and artificial flavoring, due to its intense aroma and taste, although usually in much lower concentrations.

CLOVES WELLNESS

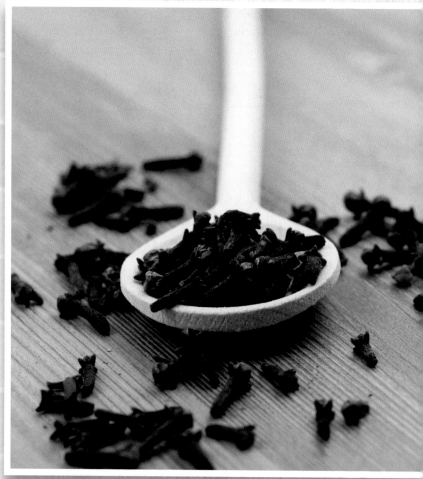

Soothe a toothache

TREAT TOOTHACHES

A toothache is painful, distracting, and if it gets bad enough it can leave you unable to get anything done until it goes away. For some quick relief, try chewing on a clove or some ground clove powder, and letting it cover the problem tooth for up to thirty minutes at a time. Cloves contain eugenol, which is known to have pain-fighting properties, so you should start to feel the results surprisingly quickly. For more intense toothaches, you can use a mortar and pestle to crush several fresh cloves, then apply the powder directly to the tooth.

ANTIMUTAGENIC PROPERTIES

Scientists have found that clove extracts are helpful in preventing diseases that are caused by cellular mutations, such as sickle cell anemia and cancer. These extracts can help cause abnormal cells to die before they can replicate, reducing your risk of tumors and disease without actually harming any normal cells.

TREAT ACNE

Eugenol, the chemical compound found in the oil of cloves, is also known for its antibacterial properties. This compound can kill the bacteria that causes acne naturally and without causing as much irritation as many of the medications that are sold in stores. A simple and easy face mask can be made using cloves to help combat acne. Just mix 5 drops clove essential oil with ¼ cup aloe vera gel and apply to any affected areas. This mask can be left on overnight for best results, or left on for 30 minutes and then rinsed off with cool water

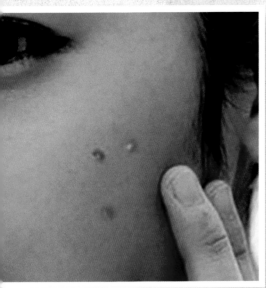

if you're in a hurry. The aloe vera gel will work in tandem with the clove oil to moisturize and soothe your skin.

Tip: Be sure to keep the mask in a dark colored container, as too much exposure to sunlight can cause it to become ineffective.

Treat acne

IMPROVE DIGESTION

Eating ground cloves helps your body produce the enzymes that it needs to digest food healthily. If you have a sensitivity to strong, spicy, or heavy foods, cloves will help you digest them without the discomfort of an upset stomach later. By helping you digest food more easily, cloves can also help you absorb more nutrition from the food you eat, letting you get more nutritional value out of every meal and reducing your chances of developing long-term digestive disorders. The easiest way to add cloves to your regular diet is to mix crushed or ground cloves into your tea, coffee, or food whenever have a meal.

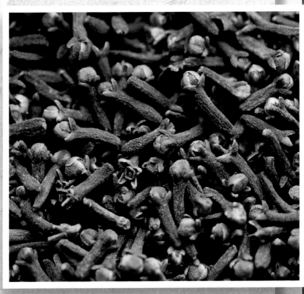

Promote healthy digestion

CLOVES WELLNESS

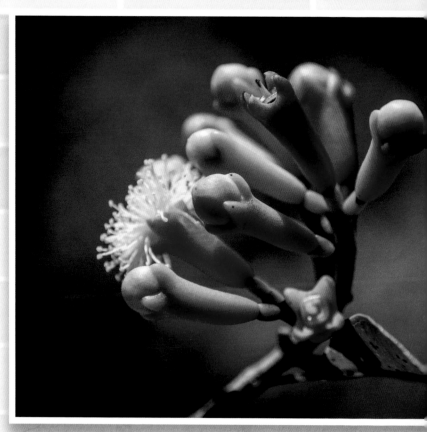

Wild cloves

ANTIBACTERIAL

Clove extracts have strong antibacterial and antiseptic properties, which can help you reduce the risk of infections, transferable diseases, and fungal infections. They are especially useful at preventing the transmission of cholera, as well as a vast number of other diseases.

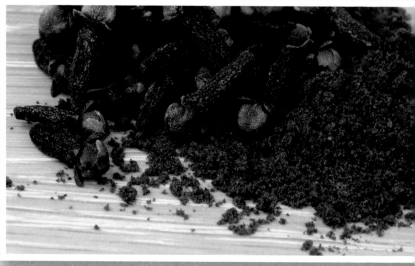

Kill bacteria

BONE HEALTH

Osteoporosis and other conditions that weaken or damage your bone density can have devastating impacts on your health and mobility. Cloves and clove extract have been shown to improve your bone density and keep your bones from becoming weak or brittle.

LIVER HEALTH

Cloves are also rich in antioxidants, which allow your body to reduce the proliferation of free radicals before they can cause much harm. Ridding your body of free radicals will slow the aging process noticeably, as well as increasing the health of every organ. The main purpose of your liver is to filter and detoxify your blood, and so by allowing the antioxidants in cloves to do some of that work, you'll be putting your liver under less stress, ensuring that your liver stays healthy and efficient for years to come.

DIABETES PREVENTION

Another way to avoid developing diabetes is to add a healthy amount of cloves to your diet. When digested, cloves act in a similar way to the insulin produced naturally by your body. This means that they are able to help keep your blood sugar down, reducing your risk of diabetes. As always, this is not a replacement for prescribed medicine, but a supplemental way to help you avoid contracting diabetes.

FIGHT INFLAMMATION

The active ingredient in cloves, eugenol, has been shown to reduce inflammation. Clove essential oil works even better for this purpose, as it gets rid of the parts of cloves that aren't as useful and increase the concentration

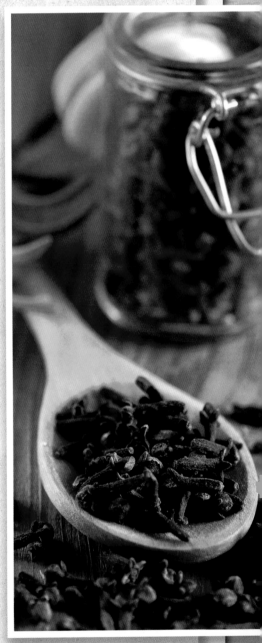

Avoid diabetes

CLOVES WELLNESS

of eugenol. Clove oil is just as readily available as regular cloves, and not especially expensive. You can apply clove oil topically to any inflamed areas—for example, rubbing clove essential oil on your knuckles can help reduce the pain of arthritis, or you can apply it to your feet after a long day spent standing up.

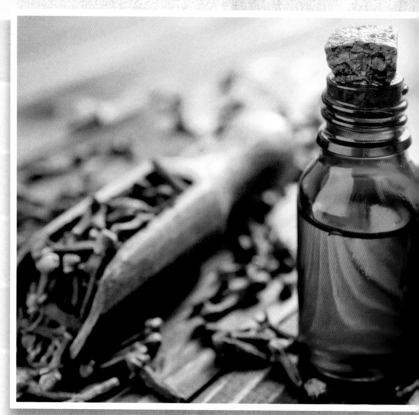

Clove essential oil

TREAT HEADACHES

As a natural anti-inflammatory, cloves are great for helping dull the pain of a headache. Most headaches are caused by inflammation or swelling of the brain to some extent, and by reducing that swelling, cloves will in turn reduce the pain you feel. For best results, try dissolving ground cloves into a large glass of water. This will have the added benefit of hydrating you, and—as the majority of headaches are caused in part by dehydration—treating the headache at its source and preventing future headaches. You might also want to try inhaling steam infused with a few drops of clove essential oil. This will be especially effective for headaches caused by allergies or clogged sinuses, and the scent of cloves will help relax you, which may ease the pain of stress-related headaches.

AID DIABETES TREATMENT

Many people who suffer from diabetes have reported lower glucose levels after regularly taking cloves. Cloves act on your body in a similar way to insulin, and can help your body be more receptive to insulin when you take diabetes medicine.

Cloves also contain a chemical compound called nigericin. Nigericin is capable of promoting your body's ability to produce insulin, and also improves cell health. You should always consult your doctor before taking cloves medicinally, especially if you are diabetic and receiving treatment.

PROMOTE DIGESTIVE HEALTH

Stomach ulcers are painful, hard to cure, and can make it difficult to enjoy your food. Cloves are capable of reducing the inflammation and pain of a stomach ulcer, as well as helping to kill any harmful bacteria that might be causing the ulcer in the first place. Eugenol also helps promote the production and health of the mucous membranes that line the walls of your stomach, which can help keep you from developing further ulcers.

IMPROVE RESPIRATORY HEALTH

Clove essential oil is great at treating any respiratory disorders like asthma and allergies. By reducing inflammation and killing bacteria, cloves can help you breathe a little more easily and ease the symptoms of these conditions. The easiest way to do this is to rub a few teaspoons of clove essential oil onto your nose and chest so that you can breathe in the oils as they evaporate, allowing your nasal passages to open up a little. Another option is to dissolve clove oil or ground cloves into a glass of hot water, which you can drink to reduce inflammation in your throat and nasal passages. For milder throat and mouth discomfort, you can simply chew a clove and keep it in your mouth for a few minutes, although this won't help much with nasal congestion.

RELIEVE STRESS

You can use clove oil to reduce stress in quite a few ways. If you're going to have a massage, you can ask your masseuse to use a clove-based massage oil, which should help relax your joints and muscles, reducing your overall stress levels. Another option is to put a few drops of essential oil in a humidifier, and either breathe some of the steam in or simply allow the clove-infused water vapor to saturate the air in the room. The scent of cloves will help you relax and you should still get some of the more concrete benefits as you breathe in the vapor.

BLACK PEPPER WELLNESS

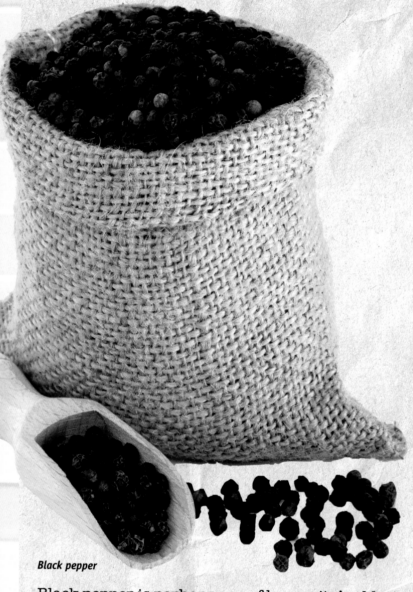

Black pepper

Black pepper is perhaps one of humanity's oldest commodities. Black peppercorns have been used as a spice and as medicine in Southeastern Asia for centuries, been buried with pharaohs in ancient Egypt, traded like currency in Europe, and now make up a larger quantity of international sales than any other spice.

Black pepper was first cultivated in India, and references to its use in food and medicine have been found in historical documents from as long ago as 2000 BC. It was so prized for its medicinal benefits and unique flavor that it was soon traded all throughout Asia, and then later made its way to the Roman empire and to Northern Africa, and eventually to all of Europe. Peppercorns were so valuable at one point that they were frequently referred to as "black gold," due to their

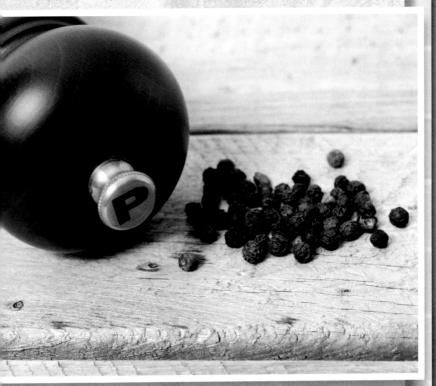

Improve digestion

common use as a form of currency, and was one of the cornerstones of the spice trade during the height of the Roman empire. By the time the seventeenth century rolled around, black pepper had become a massively-traded commodity on a global scale. Today, black pepper has spread to every corner of the world, becoming a standard requirement of any kitchen or restaurant.

When used medicinally, black pepper has a surprising number of benefits, including everything from speeding up your digestion to helping cuts heal faster. The main active ingredient in black pepper is a chemical compound known as piperine. This chemical is responsible for the signature spice of all plants in the peppercorn family, as well as many of its medicinal uses. Most significantly, piperine increases the bioavailability of other medicines, vitamins and other chemical compounds—this allows you to get the most value out of any other natural remedies you utilize, as well as man-made medicine. Piperine also lends black pepper its antibacterial properties, which can help fight off infections and kill harmful bacteria.

BLACK PEPPER WELLNESS

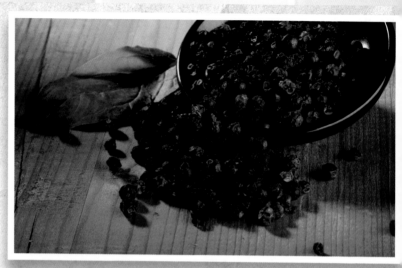

Speed up your metabolism

IMPROVE METABOLISM

Black pepper is a great metabolic aid. It helps your stomach produce stomach acid at a faster rate, which will help you digest food faster and avoid upset stomachs. A diet that includes large quantities of black pepper will help you avoid most kinds of stomach problems that result from poor digestion, and will also ensure that you get the most vitamins and nutrients from everything you eat.

RESPIRATORY AID

Black pepper is well known for its ability to make you sneeze if it gets in your nose. While, most of the time, this wouldn't exactly be desirable, it can actually be a great way to relieve congestion caused by allergies, colds, or sinus infections. A few strong sneezes can help dislodge the mucus that is over-produced by colds and allergies, relieving pressure in your sinuses and clearing out your nasal passages to let you breathe more easily.

INCREASES BIOAVAILABILITY OF OTHER MEDICINES

Eating lots of black pepper increases the bioavailability of most prescribed and over-the-counter medicines. Bioavailability, simply put, is a measure of how well the chemicals and nutrients of medicine are absorbed into your body, and how effective that medicine is once you absorb it. Higher bioavailability means that you will get the best results out of whatever medicine or vitamin supplements you take, and won't be tempted to take more than the recommended dosage if you don't feel it working right away.

FLU REMEDY

Because of its antibacterial properties, black pepper is a good way to treat a flu. While you should absolutely still consult a doctor if you get sick, adding black pepper to your diet is a good way to kill off any of the bacteria that might be making you sick.

SOOTHE SORE JOINTS AND MUSCLES

You can add ground black peppercorn—or black pepper essential oil—to a mixture of coconut oil and any other essential oils of your choice to make a soothing ointment for sore and aching joints and muscles. Simply mix the oils together into a smooth paste and massage it into your knees, hands, or any other affected areas, and you should feel some of the pain start to go away within a few minutes.

Tip: Try adding some rosemary essential oil, as it pairs nicely with the smell of black pepper and has its own soothing properties.

Use as a flu remedy

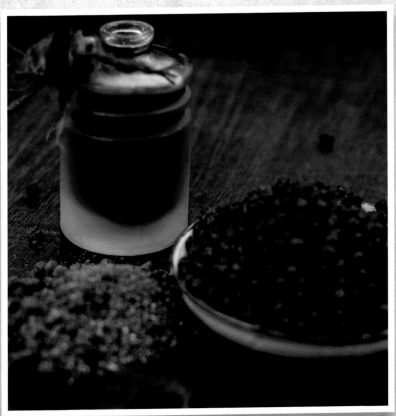

Soothe muscle pain

BLACK PEPPER WELLNESS

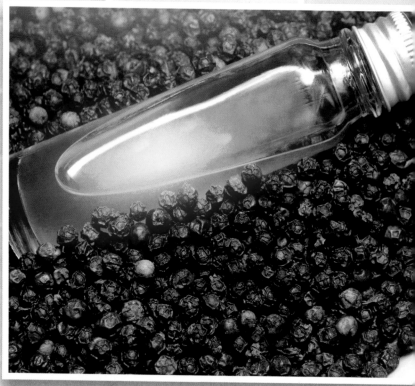

Black pepper essential oil

HEAL A CUT

This is a trick that's been around since World War II. A generous amount of finely ground black pepper can be used to slow the bleeding of a mild or moderately sized cut. Make sure to wash the cut with clean water and dry it with a clean cloth, then coat the wound in a layer of black pepper. The bleeding will begin to slow soon enough. Don't try this if your cut is worse than a surface level injury, as you might end up causing too much irritation to the wound, and always seek medical attention for a serious injury.

HELP AN UPSET STOMACH

If you have a sensitive stomach, you might regularly experience an upset stomach after an especially rich or heavy meal. One of the causes of this discomfort is that your stomach isn't ready to digest a large amount of food when you start eating. You can avoid this by eating a teaspoon or so of ground black pepper before your meal, to kickstart your stomach's production of hydrochloric acid before you actually start eating. If you don't want to eat raw black pepper, you can try mixing with something simple such as peanut butter or some crackers.

EXFOLIATION

If you struggle with dry and itchy skin, you can add black pepper to your next face or body scrub to exfoliate your skin until it feels smooth and rejuvenated. Due to is naturally anti-inflammatory and antibacterial nature—as well as the exfoliating qualities of any coarse-ground substance—black pepper is a useful way to scour any dead skin away, leaving your face looking clean and smooth once again.

TREATS DANDRUFF

Just as it can exfoliate the skin on your face, black pepper can also be used to great effect to exfoliate your scalp. To help treat dandruff, try mixing a few tablespoons black pepper with ½ tablespoon yogurt or coconut oil, and massage it gently into your scalp. Do this for at least a minute or two, and then rinse thoroughly with cool or warm water. Follow up with a gentle moisturizing conditioner for best results, and repeat this 2–3 times a week to keep your scalp healthy and free of oil and dead skin.

PROMOTES HAIR GROWTH

If you're looking to grow out your hair fast—maybe you're recovering from hair loss, a bad haircut, or just impatient to try out a new look— black pepper might be what you're after. Combine two tablespoons fresh lemon juice, one tablespoon black pepper, and (optionally) 1 teaspoon coconut oil in a jar. Apply the mixture to your scalp and leave it there for up to 30 minutes at a time, then wash your hair thoroughly with cool water. If you try this a few times a week, you should see your hair start to grow much faster than usual, and it will most likely be healthier to boot.

RELIEVE GAS

Black pepper is well known for its ability to relieve discomfort caused by gas and bloating. It helps to break down and absorb some of the gasses in your stomach—similar to the way activated charcoal works— which relieves the pressure that causes stomach aches, bloating, and general discomfort. All you need to do is add a generous helping of black pepper to your meals, but you can also eat some ground peppercorns straight if you don't mind the spiciness.

BLACK PEPPER WELLNESS

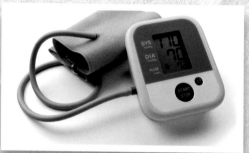

Regulate blood pressure

LOWERS BLOOD PRESSURE

Black pepper gets is signature flavor from a chemical compound called piperine, which it contains in significant quantities. This compound has been shown to reduce blood pressure when administered orally, which can help you avoid a whole slew of dangerous heart conditions. It has also been suggested that black pepper can increase your body's receptiveness to the chemical compound curcumin, a powerful blood-thinner found primarily in turmeric and ginger.

RELIEVES COLD AND COUGH

This is one of the oldest recorded uses for black pepper, and still holds up to this day. Eating black pepper can help your body fight bacteria,

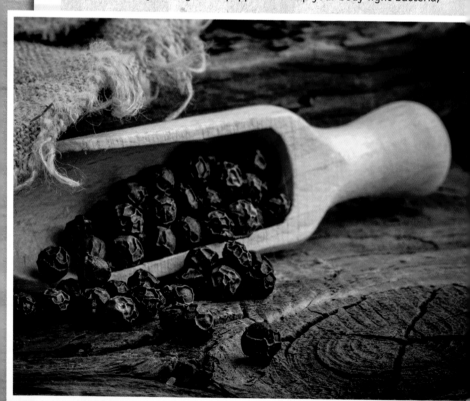

Fight a cold

promote the development of mucous membranes, and even improve your circulation. A liberal amount of black pepper in your meals should help speed up the recovery process, helping you get over a cold faster and minimizing your symptoms in the meantime. For a more direct cold and cough remedy, try combining some finely-ground black pepper with 1–2 tablespoons honey, then adding to a mug of boiling water to make a tea. You can also add some ginger and lemon juice for a little more of a boost. Two or three cups of this drink a day should clear out even the most severe cold in just a few days.

ANTIOXIDANTS

Black pepper is another household item that has strong antioxidant properties, meaning it is capable of ridding your body of free radicals and slowing down the process of aging. In fact, black pepper has one of the highest antioxidant counts of all other foods. This boost to your diet can help keep your internal organs from beginning to degrade as you grow older, avoid the development of wrinkles and skin discoloration, and keep your immune system strong.

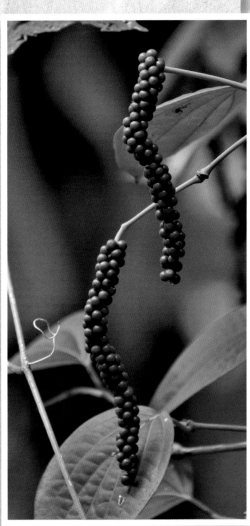
High in antioxidants

PROMOTES WEIGHT LOSS

Piperine has a number of other useful benefits outside of lowering blood pressure and adding flavor to your food. It has been shown to assist in keeping your body from storing more energy than necessary as fat, which should help you lose weight in the long run by burning through calories more efficiently instead of turning them into fat straight away. That, combined with the fact that there are barely any calories in black pepper, makes it a cheap and healthy way to add some flavor and power to your next diet. Because it has such a strong taste, you can also use black pepper as a replacement for heavier, less healthy dressings and condiments, which will also help you lose weight.

BLACK PEPPER WELLNESS

Promote healthy gums

IMPROVE MOUTH AND GUM HEALTH

If you're experiencing the discomfort of a toothache or gum infection, black pepper is a good way to get some quick relief from the pain while also fighting off the bacteria that causes these infections in the first place. Black pepper will reduce the inflammation in your gums, kill some of the harmful bacteria that might be present, and reduce some of the pain right off the bat. Try mixing 1 teaspoon salt and 1 teaspoon pepper with 1 cup warm water and swish it around your mouth for a minute or two, or use only 1 teaspoon of water and rub the mixture directly onto your gums. Clove essential oil will also work well to kill the pain and reduce inflammation.

Promote brain health

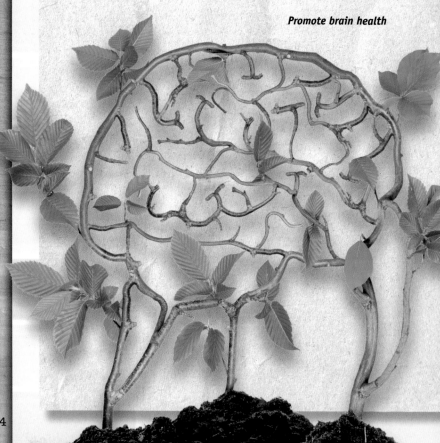

ENHANCE BRAIN HEALTH

If you're worried about the future—or present—of your mental health, you might want to start incorporating black pepper into your diet. Piperine, the primary chemical compound found in black pepper, has been shown to act similarly to a serotonin reuptake inhibitor: it restricts the function of an enzyme known as monoamine oxidase, which is primarily used to break down serotonin and reabsorb it into the body. By reducing the amount of serotonin—a chemical that helps your brain make you feel calmer and happier—that is broken down, you allow your brain to spend more time processing the serotonin and experiencing its effects. Monoamine oxidase also breaks down melatonin, which is the hormone responsible for controlling your sleep cycle. Getting enough sleep is vital for maintaining your brain's health, and can help reduce your chances of experience anxiety and depression.

Black pepper has also been shown to improve your brain's nervous system, strengthening neural pathways and preventing the buildup of plaque and the decay of neurons that can eventually lead to Alzheimer's disease. It also strengthens the cells that make up your brain, keeping them from dying too early and aiding their reproduction.

There are even some suggestions that black pepper can treat some of the symptoms of Parkinson's disease. As with monoamine oxidase, black pepper also inhibits the function of another enzyme that breaks down dopamine. Dopamine works on the brain similarly to serotonin, and has been found to be lacking in the brains of those who suffer from Parkinson's. By keeping your brain from wasting dopamine unnecessarily, you can help avoid or limit the symptoms of Parkinson's disease to some extent. Of course, you should always consult with your doctor before turning to any homeopathic medicine.

IMPROVE FERTILITY IN MEN

For those looking to start a family, black pepper can be a useful way to improve your chances. The chemicals found in black pepper—notably zinc and magnesium—have been shown to increase testosterone levels in men, improving sperm production and overall fertility rates.

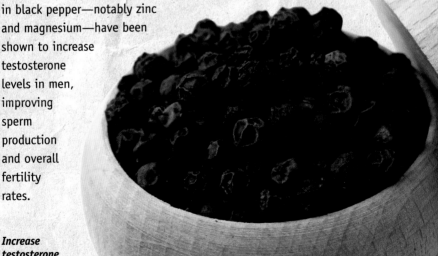

*Increase
testosterone*

BLACK PEPPER WELLNESS

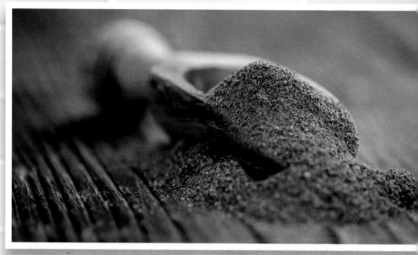

Quit smoking

HELP QUIT SMOKING

In recent years, it has become more and more commonly known that smoking is a dangerous and expensive habit that can stain your teeth, skin, hair and clothes, cause chronic lung disorders, and puts you at severe risk for lung, mouth and throat cancer. Still, knowing the risk is only part of the effort it takes to stop smoking—nicotine is one of the most addictive, most readily available drugs we use, and it can be impossible for some people to stop without some outside help. Some smokers have found that breathing in steam infused with black pepper essential oil helps reduce both nicotine cravings and withdrawal symptoms when trying to quit. Part of the reason this works is purely psychological, as the act of breathing in the vapor satisfies the desire to smoke, while the black pepper helps soothe your lungs, reducing inflammation and helping you relax.

Fight wrinkles

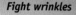

FIGHT WRINKLES

Black pepper is high in antioxidants, which indirectly contribute to keeping your skin looking young and healthy. Antioxidants limit the proliferation of free radicals in your body, and—as free radicals are largely responsible for the breakdown of elastin in your skin, causing wrinkles—getting enough antioxidants can slow down the visible aging process a great deal. Wrinkles, crow's-feet, and liver spots can all be credited to the effects of free radicals, and while you can not halt the signs of aging entirely, you can certainly avoid presenting them before your time.

The easiest way to get results is to add black pepper to every meal you eat, so that you build up a persistent buffer of antioxidants. You can also try taking 1 teaspoon black pepper with some honey, coconut oil, or water for a more direct route.

TREAT VITILIGO

Vitiligo—a skin condition that causes random patches of your skin to lose pigmentation over time—is difficult to treat, and many of the currently available treatments involve uncomfortable or even harmful chemical treatments in an attempt to restore your skin to a uniform shade. Vitiligo is relatively harmless—

Treat vitiligo

the main negative impact comes from social stigma and the judgment of others, which can have severe effects on one's mental health. Some people who have experienced vitiligo have reported that black pepper—specifically piperine, the primary chemical compound active in black pepper—can encourage skin to produce the pigmentation that is normally absent. This is a healthy, safe way to treat the symptoms of vitiligo without exposing yourself to harsh or expensive chemicals.

WARNING!

Vitiligo can occur as a symptom of other, more dangerous conditions such as hyperthyroidism and anemia, so make sure to contact your doctor regardless of the treatment you choose to follow.

REVITALIZE HAIR

To return dry, frizzy, or flat hair to its ideal volume and shine, combine 1 tablespoon each of lemon juice, finely ground black peppercorn, and coconut oil. Massage this mixture into your hair and scalp, working it from your roots outwards, and leave it in for up to twenty minutes before rinsing thoroughly with cool or lukewarm water. Repeat this a few times a week for best results, and you should start seeing your hair return to its former health in no time.

Black pepper seeds

BORAX HOME

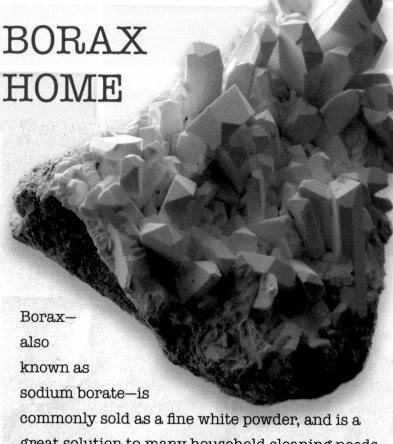

Borax—
also
known as
sodium borate—is
commonly sold as a fine white powder, and is a
great solution to many household cleaning needs.
It was first discovered centuries ago in Tibet,
where dry lake beds are home to large deposits of
borax in its colorless, crystalline form.

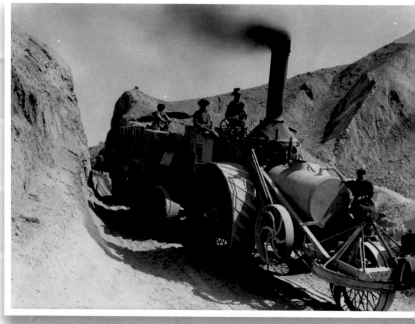

Hauling borax at Death Valley, around 1904

In the 8th century, it was traded heavily on the Silk Road. Originally, borax was first used to help extract silver and gold from raw ore, a purpose it still occasionally serves today. For the most part—especially

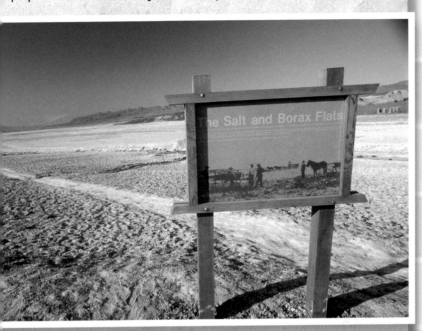

Salt and borax flats, Death Valley, California

since its discovery in other locations such as Death Valley in the 1700s—borax has been used as an all-purpose cleaning agent that is gentle enough to avoid causing damage to whatever you're cleaning, cheap enough to use liberally on just about everything, and powerful enough to wash away dirt and grime from most surfaces. While borax is generally found in salt deposits and the evaporated floors of seasonal lakes, it has also become common practice to produce synthetic, man-made borax.

This simple substance can be used to clean tiles, keep out pests like mice and fleas, and even dissolve rust. If you're looking for a natural and inexpensive way to keep your home clean, healthy, and free of harsh cleaning chemicals, try using borax as a quick and effective all-purpose cleaner.

WARNING!
Be sure to consult with your vet and/or doctor before using borax to clean carpets, floors, or any other areas where children or pets might be able to ingest it accidentally, as borax is not edible and may be toxic to children and small animals.

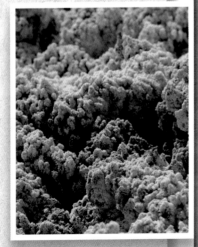

Borax crystals in raw form on the ground

BORAX HOME

CARPET CLEANING

Borax is a powerful and inexpensive cleaning agent. Give a boost to the cleaning power of your carpet cleaning machine by adding ½ cup borax per gallon of water in your reservoir. Alternately, you can mop your floors by dissolving ½ cup borax in 1 gallon warm water in a bucket before cleaning.

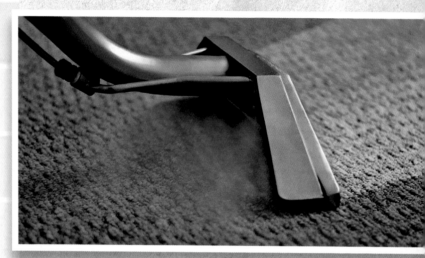

Clean carpets

KEEP OUT PESTS

If you are dealing with an infestation of roaches or ants, you can use borax to eliminate the problem. Simply make a mixture of equal parts sugar and borax and sprinkle the mixture anywhere you think the insects may be entering your home.

Fight infestations

TOILET BOWL CLEANER

For an easy way to keep your toilet clean, try using borax. Before going to bed, pour 1 cup borax into the bowl of your toilet. Let it sit overnight; when you wake up, give the toilet bowl a good scrub with a toilet brush. The borax will loosen any grime deposits to make cleaning your toilet a breeze. Be sure to keep the lid of the toilet closed overnight to prevent your pets from ingesting any borax.

Clean toilets

FLEA KILLER

If you suspect that you have fleas,
try using borax to eliminate the problem.
Identify any and all areas where you
suspect that fleas are hatching and sprinkle
a light layer of borax over the area. Let the
borax sit on the area for a day and vacuum
the borax away. Good places to check are dog beds,
carpets, and any other upholstered area in your home.

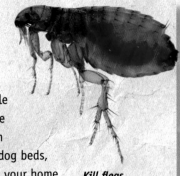

Kill fleas

MICE DETERRENT

In order to counter any
unwelcome mice visitors,
sprinkle borax on the
floor along the walls
and on any areas
where you believe the
mice may be entering your home. Mice

Keep mice away tend to run along the floor at the base of walls but
dislike getting borax on their feet and therefore are less likely to return
to that area of the house.

WARNING!
Be sure to move pet beds to a safe place while treating.

PRESERVING FLOWERS

Dried flowers make a beautiful decorative addition to any home. While drying flowers in the traditional method works, it does not eliminate the possibility of wilting. By using borax, you can ensure the quality

Preserve flowers

of your dried flowers. Borax will remove any moisture from blossoms and leaves which will prevent any wilting that may normally occur. Make a mixture of one part borax with two parts cornmeal and sprinkle the bottom of a shoebox with the mixture. Take any variety of fresh flower and lay it in the box and sprinkle the remaining borax and cornmeal mixture over the flowers. Close the shoebox and store in a cool, dry place for two weeks until your flowers are completely dry.

BORAX HOME

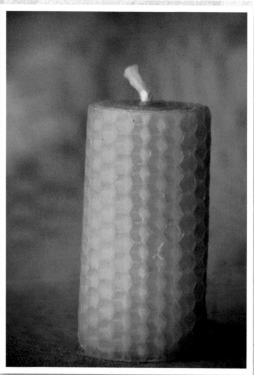

Make your own candles

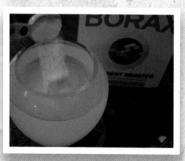

Remove sticker residue

BETTER HOMEMADE CANDLES

While making your beeswax candles, try treating your wicks with borax. In a glass of warm water, combine 1 teaspoon salt and 1 teaspoon borax and stir until dissolved. Soak the wicks you plan on using for your candles in the solution. Doing so will reduce ash production and any smoke problems while burning your homemade candles.

RESIDUE REMOVER

If you've ever tried to remove a sticker and found a sticky, unsightly smear of adhesive left behind, you already know how difficult removing that residue can be. Luckily, you can use borax as an easy way to dissolve the gooey substance left behind in just a few minutes. Mix together two parts borax and one part water in a cup, soak a clean washcloth with the solution, and rub it into the adhesive for thirty seconds or so to remove any lingering traces of adhesive.

CLEANING COOKWARE

Borax is a cheap, efficient, and gentle cleaning solution for just about any surface or utensil in your kitchen, from a ceramic plate to a nonstick frying pan. All you need to do is sprinkle powdered borax onto whatever needs cleaning and scrub for a few seconds with a damp,

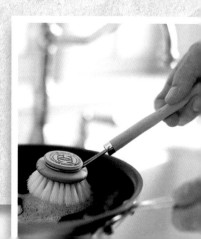

clean cloth, and any stains or food residue should wipe away easily. Rinse the surface thoroughly with water once you're done, of course, as borax should be assumed to be as inedible as any other soap.

REFRIGERATOR DEODORIZER

A simple fact of life when one owns a refrigerator is that, given enough time without regular cleaning, your fridge will eventually start to smell. You can use borax to clean up spilled food, stains, or simply wipe down the shelves of your fridge to rid it of any lingering unpleasant odors. Soak a sponge in a bowl or jug filled with 1 tablespoon borax and 1 quart hot water, and use it to clean any surface in your

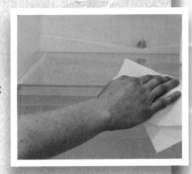

Clean your fridge

fridge that has becomes stained or discolored. Wipe the shelves clean with a damp cloth afterwards, and then dry with a clean paper towel.

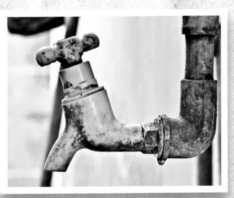

Scour rust

REMOVE RUST

Rust is one of the most common and most unsightly occurrences in a home, especially if you live in a humid environment or use metal utensils and tools that aren't already rust-resistant. To get any rusty metal shining like it's brand new again, mix 2 tablespoons borax, 1 tablespoon lemon juice, and ½ tablespoon or so of water in a cup. You may need to add more or less water, depending on how much you need to make a smooth paste. Spread the resulting soap-like paste onto any rusty areas, leave on for up to 30 minutes at a time depending on the severity of the rust, and then scrub clean with a coarse sponge.

CLEAN MATTRESSES

Borax is an excellent cleaning agent for removing just about any kind of stains from a mattress, whether you spill a glass of wine, a pet pees on your bed, or the white fabric has simply become discolored after years of use. First, apply a damp cloth to the affected area. Thoroughly rub in powdered borax, and vacuum up any remaining residue after the paste dries.

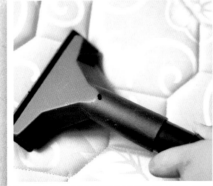

Clean your mattress

BORAX HOME

SHOWER, TUB, & TILE

Showers walls and tiles can be tricky things to clean. If you use too harsh of a cleaning solution, you can strip away patterns or colors in ceramic tiles, or even scratch through a glaze or ceramic finish, leaving ugly and hard to replace marks. To keep your ceramics and tiles spotless and unmarred, coat a wet sponge with a layer of powdered borax and use it to clean any bathroom surfaces. Borax grains are generally fine enough to avoid leaving scratches on even the most malleable materials, while still washing away dirt and debris.

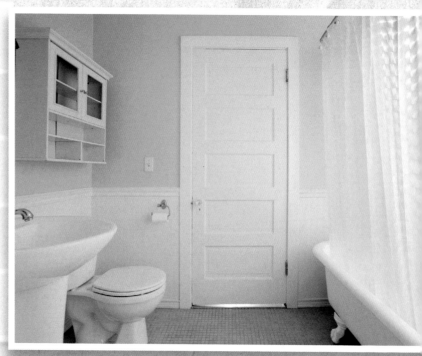

Clean your bathroom

CLEAN HUMIDIFIERS

Humidifiers need to be regularly maintained to keep them from starting to smell. With the amount of water that passes through them on a constant basis, it's easy for parts of your humidifier to start to smell of mildew or stagnant water. To make sure your humidifier is running as clean as the day you got it, fill the tank with 1 gallon water mixed with ½ cup borax,

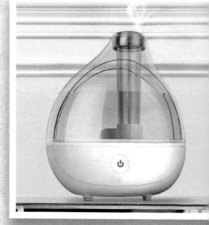

Deodorize humidifiers

and run the humidifier as normal for twenty minutes or so. Remove the tank and dump out the excess water and borax, rinse it clean, and then you can go back to using your humidifier normally. If you like, you also add a little lemon juice or a few drops of an essential oil of your choice, which should make the whole room smell a little nicer while you clean your humidifier.

OUTDOOR FURNITURE

Outdoor furniture is pretty easy to clean for the most part, but you want to be careful what kind of cleaner you use. Anything involving bleach or especially harsh chemicals can cause color fading or can strip off waterproofing that keeps your outdoor furniture from getting damaged when it rains. Borax is gentle enough to keep your furniture in good condition while still

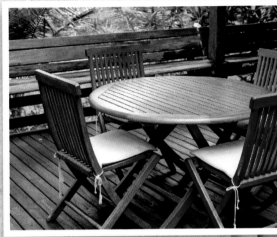

Clean outdoor furniture

scouring away dirt, dust, and any other accumulated grime. The easiest way to clean your furniture with borax is to mix 2 tablespoons borax and 1 quart warm water in a spray bottle. Use this to spray down your furniture, then wipe all surfaces dry with a clean cloth. You can also add a little lemon juice to the bottle for some extra strength cleaning.

GARBAGE CAN DEODORIZER

To keep a garbage can clean—and to keep your house from smelling bad even when the garbage can is empty—fill a garbage can with water and 1 cup powdered borax. Leave it to soak for a few hours to completely eliminate odors, then rinse clean. In order to prevent odors from reappearing and keep bugs away, sprinkle borax after it's clean. If your trash can isn't water-tight, you can use more borax than water to make a paste and apply it liberally to the inside of the trash can. Leave this for a few hours and then rinse clean for the same deodorizing effect.

UNCLOG DRAINS

If your kitchen sink or bathroom drain is clogged, you're most likely going to want to fix that problem as soon as possible. A clogged drain can lead to flooding, can make your bathroom

BORAX HOME

or kitchen smell bad, and generally make it impossible to use whatever feature the drain is connected to until the clog is gone. An easy way to clear out a clogged drain is to mix ½ cup borax into 2 cups boiling water. Pour the solution into the drain—slowly, to avoid it overflowing or scalding you with hot water—and leave it there for twenty minutes. Then, simply run the water for 2–3 minutes to finish rinsing away any residual clogs. The combination of hot water and borax should be more than enough to dissolve even stubborn bloackages.

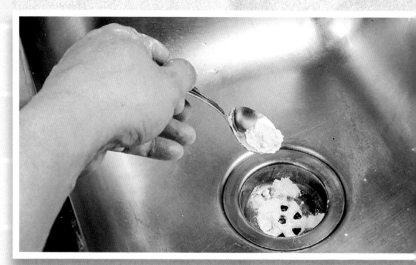

Unclog drains

GARBAGE DISPOSAL CLEANER

A garbage disposal can quickly start to smell if you don't take measures to keep it clean. To keep old food debris and other residue from building up and making your kitchen smell like rotting food, all you need to do is dump a few tablespoons of borax powder down the drain. Let the powder sit for an hour or so without running the tap, and then run hot water for a few minutes. This should wash away any accumulated grime that might cause unpleasant odors. Repeat this process whenever your garbage disposal starts to smell, and you should never have to worry about keeping it clean again.

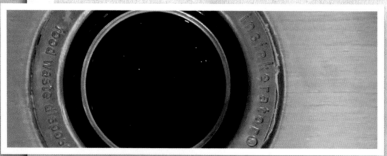

Clean garbage disposal

KILL WEEDS

Borax is a powerful weed killer and can be applied to concrete cracks and walkways where weeds normally grow. Mix two tablespoons borax into a spray bottle of water and spray liberally onto any weeds—or areas where you want to keep weeds from growing. Make sure to not use this mixture anywhere near your garden, as it will not only kill weeds, but also flowers and vegetables. Avoid spraying borax anywhere near where your pets or other animals wander, as ingesting borax can be toxic, especially for smaller animals like cats and rabbits.

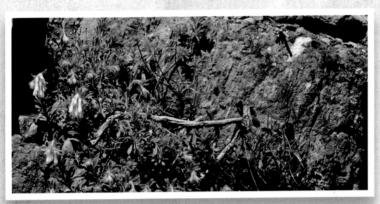

Fight weeds

SHINE CHINA

Many people have china tea sets or statuettes that have been passed down to them as family heirlooms, or that were purchased in an antique store. Old china can be valuable, impossible to replace, and of sentimental importance, which is why keeping it clean without harming it is so important. To restore old, tarnished china, soak the piece in a sink full of warm (not hot) water and ½ cup borax for a few minutes. Rinse off the solution and clean a second time with a soft cloth, and your china should shine like new.

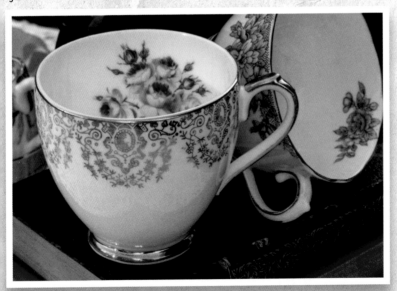

Shine china

BORAX HOME

CLEAN HAIRBRUSHES AND COMBS

Over years of use, brushes and combs can build up a surprising amount of loose hair, or can simply become unpleasantly grimy. To wash away any tangles of hair and clean your hairbrushes and combs, combine ¼ cup borax and 1 tablespoon dish soap with warm water in a large bowl. Allow your brush or comb to soak in the mixture for 1 hour, then rinse clean and allow to air dry. Any loose hair should come away easily, leaving your combs clean as the day you got them.

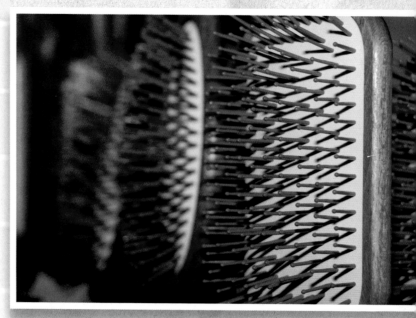

Clean brushes

MOLD INHIBITOR

If you want to keep a part of your house from becoming moldy, or if you need to get rid of mold that's already started to show up, make a thick paste of borax powder and water to apply to any desired areas. Make sure to use enough water that the solution can soak into the area thoroughly, but not so much that it runs like liquid. Allow the paste to sit until dry, which may take several hours, and then rinse the area clean and pat dry. Keep any children or pets away from this area while the borax dries, to make sure they don't ingest any borax.

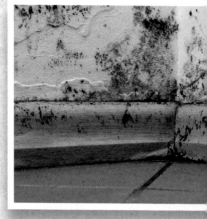

Fight mold

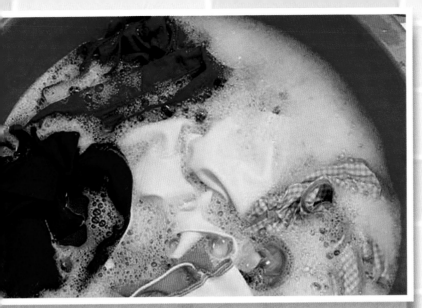

Treat fabric

MAKE CLOTHING FLAME RETARDANT

One potentially life-saving use for borax is to make clothing flame-retardant. This won't necessarily make the fabric fireproof, but it will make it much less likely to catch or spread fire when exposed to high heat. Soak clothes, drapes, or other fabric in a solution of ½ cup borax combined with 1 gallon of water, or spray non-washable clothes and allow them to air-dry. This solution will wash out of clothing over time and should be reapplied regularly to maintain effectiveness.

REFRESH LINENS

If your clothes have developed a musty smell from being left in the washing machine for too long, borax can act as a powerful restoration agent. Allow your garments to soak for two to three hours in a mixture of 2 quarts water and 2 cups borax to remove mildew and restore linens.

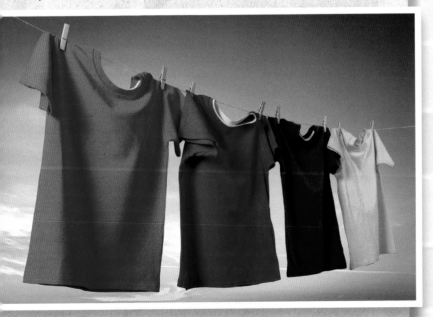

Refresh linens

GARLIC WELLNESS

Garlic is one of the most commonly used ingredients in recipes all over the world, due to its distinctive flavor, smell, and ability to bring out the flavors of every other ingredient in a dish. Similarly to its many uses as a culinary ingredient, garlic also carries a surprising number of health and wellness benefits when made a primary part of your diet.

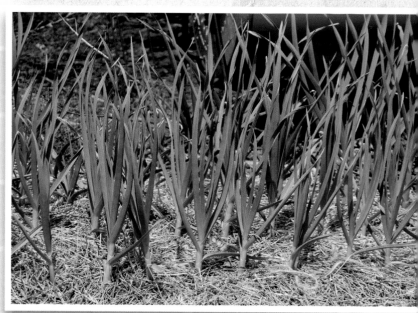

High in antioxidants

Whether cooked or eaten raw, garlic is high in antioxidants, a powerful antibacterial agent, and packed with nutritional value. You can even use it topically to fight infections, improve hair health, and relieve the pain of toothache.

Garlic is naturally found all over the world, and has been used for centuries as both a food and medicine in dozens of countries. The use of garlic has been recorded in

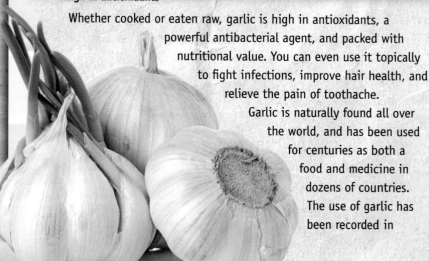

Wild garlic

ancient Egypt, Rome, Greece, and China, and was believed to convey a vast number of health benefits when eaten raw or used in food. It has been used as a preservative, offered as a religious sacrifice, traded as a commodity, and offered as a cure-all to countless illnesses over the last few thousand years. In more recent years, modern science has allowed us to look a little more deeply into what makes garlic so good for you.

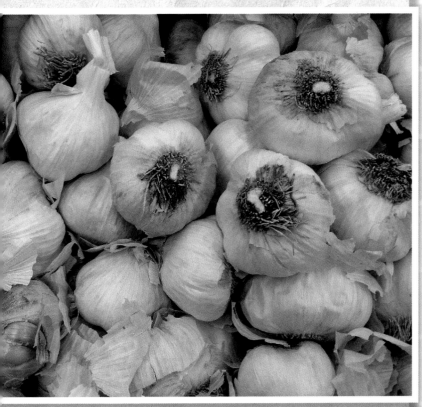

Garlic

Allicin, among several other similar sulfur compounds, is the chemical that is primarily responsible for the unique flavor, smell, and beneficial properties of garlic. Interestingly, allicin is an unstable compound; it is only released when garlic is crushed, cut, or chewed, at which point its benefits becomes readily available.

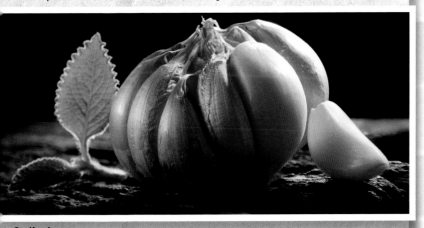

Garlic cloves

GARLIC WELLNESS

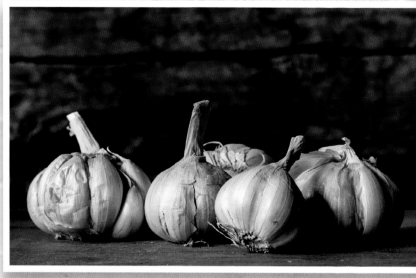

Promote skin health

TREAT ECZEMA

Eczema affects many people around the world, and while medications are available over the counter and from your doctor, natural remedies are often just as effective and come with less harmful side effects. Adding garlic to your diet can be helpful in preventing flair-ups and reducing itching caused by rashes. A paste can be made from garlic cloves to get quicker relief from your eczema symptoms. Simply grind all cloves from one head of garlic with juice from about ½ of a lemon to form a paste. Apply the paste to the affected area and allow to sit on the skin for about 30 minutes.

CLEANSE ACNE

Garlic is a surprisingly great way to kill the bacteria that causes acne, clearing up your pores and fighting breakouts. All you have to do is gently rub a cut piece of raw garlic against your skin wherever a breakout is starting for a few minutes, and the antibacterial properties of the garlic should kill off a fair amount of the bacteria and help bring down the redness and swelling.

FIGHT COLDS

Garlic is high in antioxidants, which makes it both a healthy addition to your everyday diet and also a powerful contributor to fighting off the common cold. Making a strong garlic and ginger

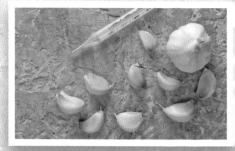

Boost your immune system

tea—perhaps with a spoonful or two of honey to improve the taste a little—is a surefire way to help keep down the symptoms of a cold, and regularly eating a decent amount of garlic should keep your immune system strong and fend off colds before they start affecting you in the first place.

REMOVE A SPLINTER

This has been used as a home remedy for centuries. In households all over the world, you've probably already been advised to use a cut piece of garlic to remove a splinter—surprisingly enough, it actually works. Securing a piece of garlic to the area just over the splinter with a bandage should soften the skin and help lift the splinter to the surface so that you can remove it more easily. Garlic is also great at killing bacteria, which should help keep the splinter from starting an infection.

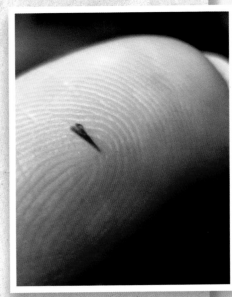

Remove splinters

REGULATE BLOOD PRESSURE

One of the key chemical compounds in garlic is called allicin. This compound helps limit the function of a peptide known as angiotensin II that causes blood vessels to contract. By reducing the contraction of blood vessels, you will allow your blood to flow more freely, which will reduce blood pressure and reduce your risk of heart attacks, blood clots, and strokes.

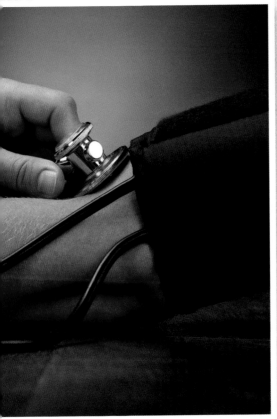

Lower blood pressure

GARLIC WELLNESS

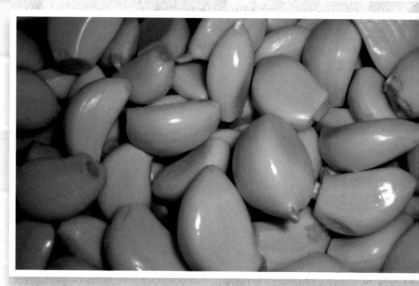

Peeled garlic

START YOUR DAY

One common practice, especially for people who struggle with sinus issues, is to simply eat a clove of raw garlic every morning. This can be a pretty harrowing experience given how strong raw garlic is, but it's sure to clear out your sinuses just as well as eating other spicy foods. It should also help wake you up thoroughly for the day ahead, as well as kick-starting your digestive system and giving you all the other health benefits that come with a diet high in garlic.

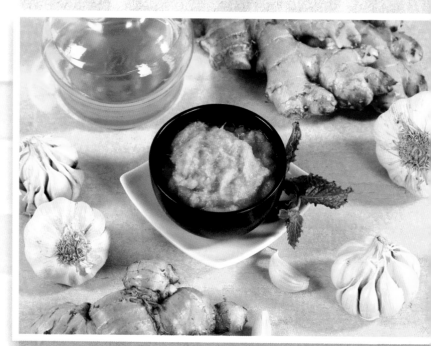

Garlic is useful in many forms

PREVENT HEART DISEASE

You can add garlic to your diet to help lower your cholesterol and minimize your risk of heart disease. Raw garlic will give you better results, but cooked garlic will still provide benefits and will be much easier to eat regularly. A diet high in garlic has been shown to reduce bad cholesterol, while

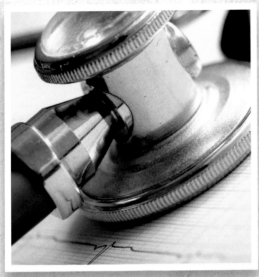

Improve heart health

also regulating your blood pressure and blood sugar levels—all of which can help you avoid heart disease.

PREVENT WRINKLES

Garlic is naturally high in antioxidants, which are your body's main defense against free radicals. Free radicals can accelerate the aging process and cause your skin to lose its elasticity, resulting in wrinkles and age spots. By introducing a higher count of antioxidants to your body, you will be able to avoid showing signs of aging prematurely, keeping your skin healthy and free of wrinkles. For a more targeted approach, you can also make a DIY mask with raw garlic. All you need to do is peel and finely crush 3 garlic cloves, add 3 tablespoons olive oil and 2 tablespoons honey, and blend together until a smooth paste is formed. Place the paste in a sealed container and refrigerate overnight. Apply the mask to your face for 15–20 minutes, then rinse it off with warm water and pat dry. This mask should be applied about three times a week for best results.

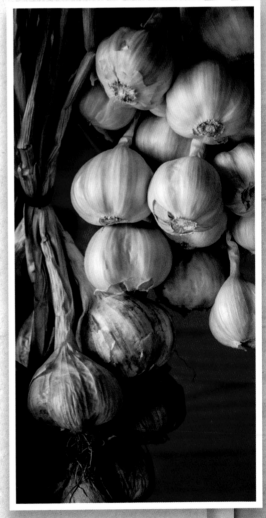

Prevent wrinkles

GARLIC WELLNESS

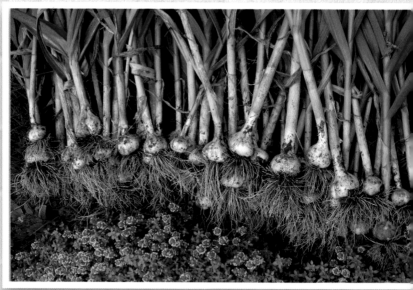

Freshly pulled garlic

REPAIR GLASS

Interestingly, garlic juice can be used to repair hairline fractures in glass and porcelain. Simply crush or grind a clove of garlic and collect the juice, and then apply it to the cracked glass to keep the damage from worsening. This works because garlic juice is a natural adhesive, forming a glue-like substance when it dries in open air.

FIGHT BACTERIA

Garlic has been used since ancient times as an effective medicine to fight against infections caused by bacteria, parasites, and fungi. Modern science has found that the chemical allicin is responsible for garlic's ability to fight against all types of infections, and that—unlike many antibiotics that are prescribed or bought over the counter—garlic will not kill the good bacteria found in your body that helps keep you healthy. To make it even easier to use garlic to fight infections, you can also make a garlic concentrate. Simply crush a few cloves of garlic and allow them to soak in olive oil for a day or two, before either consuming it in food or applying it directly to wounds to help prevent and fight infection.

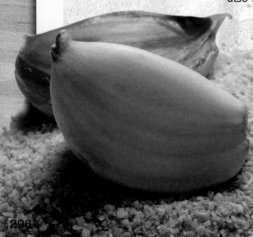

TREAT ATHLETE'S FOOT

Because garlic is so good at killing most kinds of fungus, it can be a great solution for conditions like athlete's foot. Crush up some garlic—anywhere from a few cloves to a whole head of garlic, depending on how severe your case is—and allow them to infuse in a warm foot bath. Soak your feet in this concoction for 20–30 minutes, and you should start seeing results soon enough. Try repeating this daily to make sure your athlete's foot vanishes completely.

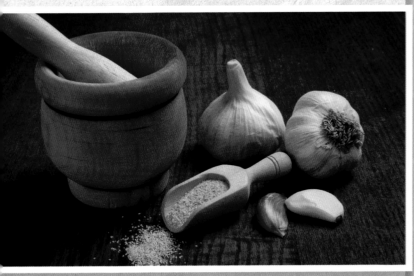

Treat athlete's foot

BONE HEALTH

While garlic is a useful way to keep just about anyone healthy, it can be especially helpful for menopausal women. This is because of its ability to increase and regulate estrogen levels, which is important to help keep bones healthy and to ward off osteoporosis. Studies have shown that adding only a small amount of garlic to your daily diet or taking it as a daily dose of raw garlic or extract significantly increased estrogen levels in menopausal women. Garlic also improves bone health for anyone who eats it regularly enough, as it contains high amounts of vitamins and minerals that help strengthen bones, such as vitamin B6, vitamin C, zinc, and manganese.

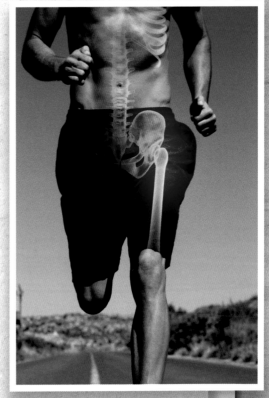

Prevent osteoporosis

GARLIC WELLNESS

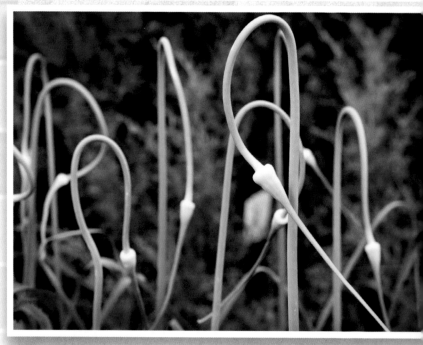

Garlic Scape

PREVENT HAIR LOSS

Garlic can be used to prevent your hair from falling out, and even to stimulate hair growth. Because it improves circulation, massaging raw garlic or garlic oil into your scalp can improve blood flow to the scalp, which will promote the growth of new hair and keep it from falling out. Garlic will also kill any bacteria or fungus that may be causing dandruff, hair loss, or damaging the health of your scalp.

TREAT PSORIASIS

Because garlic has such strong anti-inflammatory properties, it can provide a great deal of relief to those suffering from the symptoms of psoriasis. Psoriasis causes rashes of dry, itchy skin all over the body, which can be unbearably uncomfortable when left untreated. Some psoriasis patients swear by the practice of applying garlic oil to any affected areas, reducing the discomfort and redness surprisingly quickly.

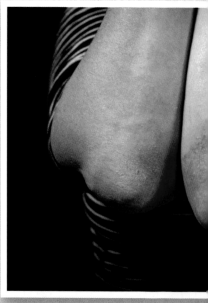

Psoriasis

LOSE WEIGHT

Losing weight can be difficult, especially when you want to change your eating habits rather than your diet itself. Garlic can help combat weight gain caused by overeating, as it convinces your brain that you're more full than you are when you eat it, keeping you from eating more than you need to. Garlic is also good for your digestive system, speeding up your metabolism a little to help you lose weight faster.

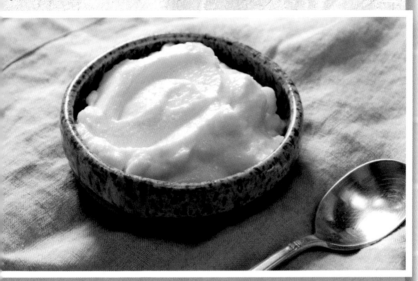

Promote weight loss

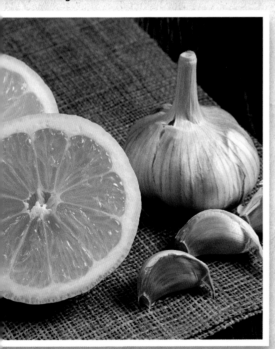

Treat a cough

TREAT A COUGH

If you have a cough or a sore throat, and find yourself lacking any kind of cough syrup, garlic tea can be a useful replacement. Boiling raw garlic in a cup of water will make a strong tea that should lower the inflammation that causes pain and irritation in your throat, as well as helping to kill bacteria that might be causing the inflammation. It might be a little hard to drink straight garlic tea on its own, of course, so feel free to add honey, ginger, and/or lemon juice to your tea.

GARLIC WELLNESS

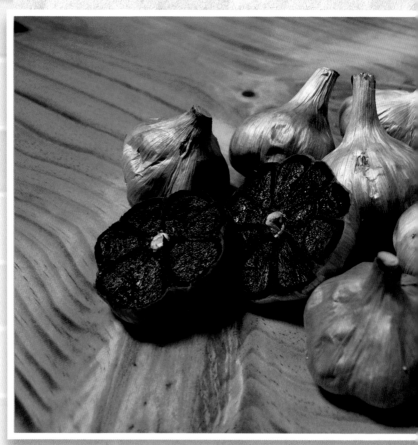

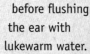

Treat ear infections

TREAT EAR INFECTIONS

Ear infections are painful, hard to treat, and make it difficult to go about your day until the discomfort is gone. Garlic excels at killing bacteria and fighting infections, which makes it an invaluable way to fight off painful, frustrating ear infections. One tried and true way to do this is to put a few drops of garlic oil in the affected ear, leaving it to soak for ten minutes or so before flushing the ear with lukewarm water.

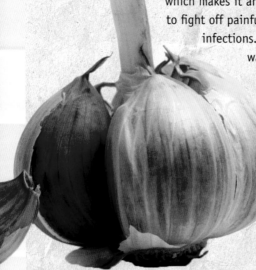

REPEL MOSQUITOS

Although you might not want to smell like garlic all day, you can use garlic oil as a surprisingly effective mosquito and insect repellant. Mix an ounce or so of garlic oil with 2 cups water and 1 teaspoon lemon juice, and use a spray bottle to apply it to your skin to keep insects away. To make your own garlic oil instead of buying it in a store, you can infuse several crushed garlic cloves into an ounce of mineral oil for several hours before pouring the resulting solution through a sieve or strainer and into a bottle.

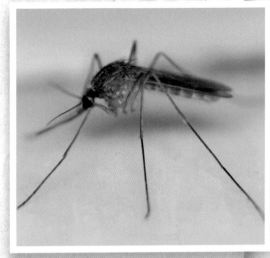

Insect repellant

GET RID OF BLACKHEADS

You can make a quick, cheap facial mask out of garlic to help remove blackheads and keep your skin looking healthy and soft. In a bowl, combine 2 finely ground or blended garlic cloves with 3 tablespoons oatmeal, 2 drops tea tree oil, and 5 drops lemon juice. Stir in 2 tablespoons honey until a smooth paste is formed, then allow the mask to sit covered overnight. Apply the mask in a thin layer and leave it on for up to 20 minutes at a time, long enough to let the garlic do its work. Rinse off with warm water, then apply a gentle moisturizer. For best results, use this mask three times a week.

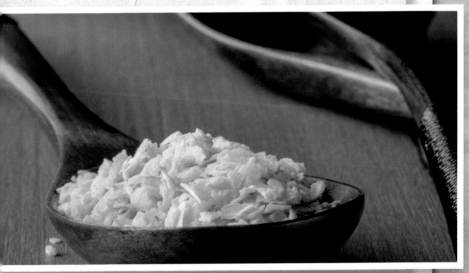

GARLIC WELLNESS

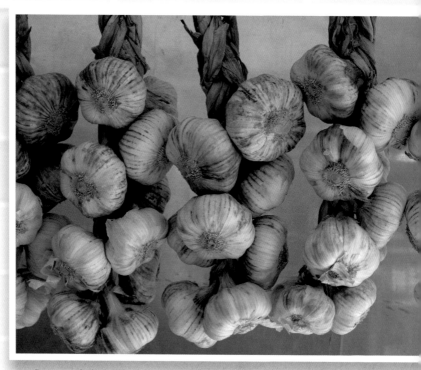

Improve cholesterol

MAINTAIN HEALTHY CHOLESTEROL LEVELS

It is claimed that the antioxidant properties of garlic offer great cardiovascular benefits, and can lower cholesterol and triglyceride levels by up to 15%. Garlic can also help with the prevention of plaque buildup on the artery walls, by countering the oxidation of low-density lipoprotein (LDL).

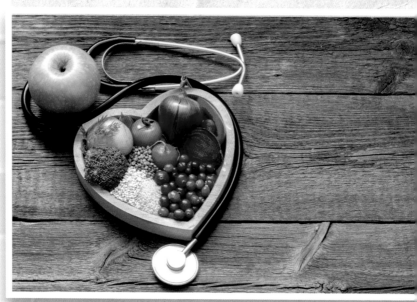

Improve blood sugar

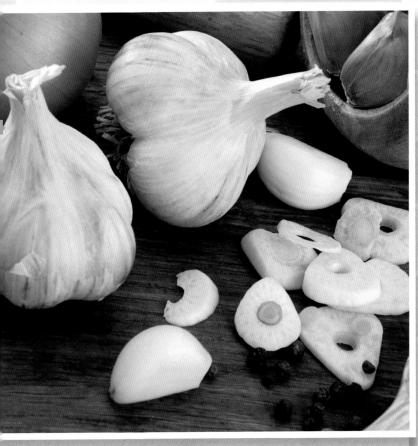

Sliced garlic

PREVENT BLOOD CLOTS

Another benefit of this miraculous allium is that it can help to prevent the formation of blood clots. Garlic contains a substance called ajoene, which has anti-clotting properties that prevent platelets from clumping together, thus reducing the risk of blood clots.

PROMOTE STABLE BLOOD SUGAR LEVELS

Another substance present in garlic—allicin—has the effect of increasing insulin secretion, which in turn slows the glycation process, which occurs in tandem with increased blood sugar. Ingesting garlic daily by adding it to your favorite meal can promote stable blood sugar levels. Consult your doctor if you have diabetes, as garlic is not a substitute for prescribed medication.

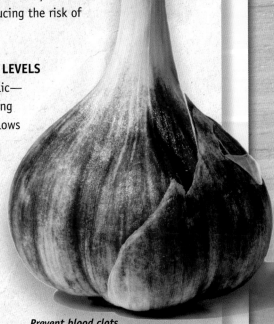

Prevent blood clots

GARLIC WELLNESS

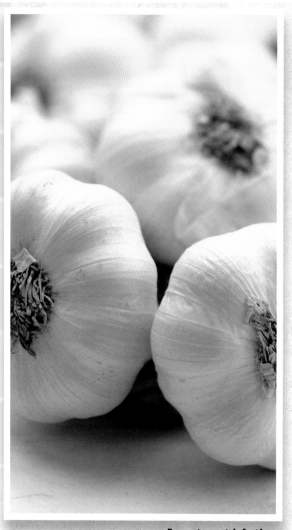

PREVENTS YEAST INFECTIONS

Given how rich garlic is in antioxidants, garlic has a very positive impact on the immune system, and protects the body from microbes such as worms, fungi and yeast—in particular, the presence of ajoene helps prevent the growth of the fungus *Candida albicans*, another form of yeast that commonly sets in when other factors weaken your immune system or digestive health.

Prevent yeast infections

ABSORB MORE MINERALS

The *Journal of Agricultural and Food Chemistry* claims that garlic can increase the body's ability to absorb zinc and iron if taken with whole grains. It also helps to increase the production of the ferro protein, which can also help increase your body's ability to absorb iron.

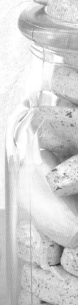

CLEANSE YOUR LIVER

Garlic can help your body get rid of unwanted toxins by activating the enzymes in the liver. Sulphur is a vital requirement in the liver's ability to detoxify toxins and harsh medications—and garlic is a great source of sulphur. Another beneficial impact on the liver is that the allicin and selenium in garlic helps to enhance bile production, which in turn has a positive impact on the symptoms of a condition known as "fatty liver."

TREAT INSECT BITES

To reduce the itching and swelling from insect bites—be it a mosquito bite or a scorpion sting—slice a garlic clove and rub the area with the sliced side. Garlic can sting, so use it with caution—only rub the garlic clove over the bite a few times. If the bite area is large, you might consider using a garlic poultice instead. To make a poultice crush two or three cloves of garlic with the back of a fork or with a garlic press. Lay out a piece of cheesecloth and double it over. Place the crushed garlic into the middle of the cheesecloth. Fold up the cheesecloth, folding two opposite sides over the garlic and then

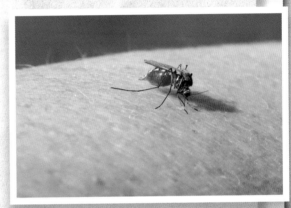

Treat insect bites

the two other sides over the top of that. Put the poultice in a bowl of warm water for about 1 minute. Squeeze out excess water and place the poultice on the bite.

TOOTHACHE

Garlic has been used for a long time in medicine to reduce the severe pain from a toothache. There are several ways to use garlic as a remedy, but one of the most popular and effective methods is to combine salt and a garlic clove to create a fine paste. Apply the paste to the affected area and rinse after several minutes to relieve pain

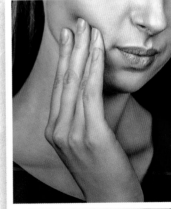

Relieve toothache

from a toothache. Be careful not to apply too much, as the garlic and salt can cause mild discomfort.

GARLIC WELLNESS

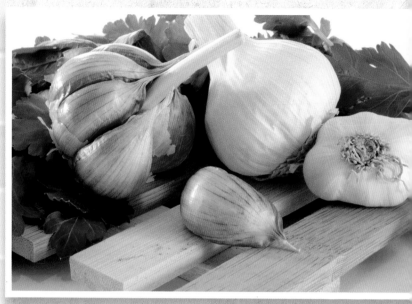

Garlic

STY REMEDY

Garlic's natural anti-inflammatory properties make it a great solution for anyone dealing with the pain and discomfort of a sty. Apply a clove of garlic directly on the sty each day to reduce the pain and swelling, as well as killing bacteria. Doing this twice a day will help relieve pain, and garlic's antibacterial properties will restore the area affected by the sty.

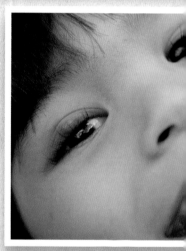

Treat a sty

GINGIVITIS

While it won't do any favors for your breath, garlic can do wonders for treating gingivitis. This condition causes the gums to swell and bleed. Chewing cloves of garlic helps to reduce gum inflammation caused by gingivitis. Continued use of garlic after a meal can help prevent symptoms from occurring due to the antibacterial properties of garlic.

BLADDER INFECTION PREVENTION

Bladder infections are caused by harmful bacteria which use the body to create bacterial colonies. By ingesting a clove of garlic or a teaspoon of garlic juice, one can kill the bacteria causing the condition. Start your day off by consuming garlic to prevent infections from reappearing.

TREAT COLD SORES

A common home remedy for dealing with cold sores is to apply crushed garlic directly to the affected area. This solution may cause mild discomfort, but it should help conquer cold sores, especially when coupled with other treatments. For example, honey has vitamins and minerals, so consider applying it to the area to speed up healing. Garlic's anti-inflammatory properties will reduce the swelling and the honey will help the wound heal much faster. In addition to treating existing cold sores, garlic can prevent cold sores from reappearing if consumed regularly.

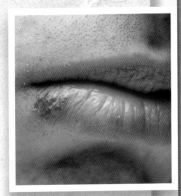

Treat cold stores

NUTRITION

Garlic contains several minerals that the body needs, such as potassium, zinc, and iron. It also contains many vitamins necessary to one's health, such as vitamin C, K, and B6. One rare compound in garlic is allicin, which has shown effectiveness in preventing the common cold and several other viral infections. Garlic is a healthy, low-calorie herb that can serve as a substitute for other unhealthy snacks.

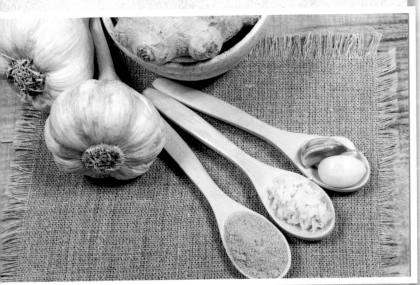

Improve nutrition

PREVENT HEAVY METAL POISONING

Heavy metals, such as lead and zinc, can poison your body from the inside and cause irreversible organ damage. Garlic can be used to prevent this due to the high amount of sulfur present in the herb. Sulfur aids the body in absorbing iron and zinc, although one should be sure to monitor the amount of heavy metals they consume and be sure to maintain a healthy diet.

GARLIC WELLNESS

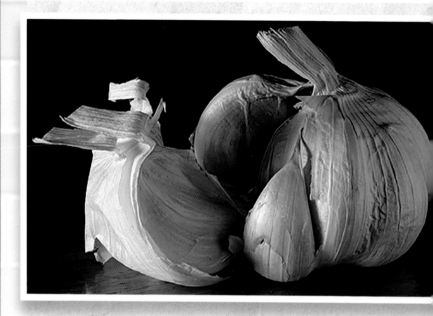

BOOST DIGESTION

Including garlic in one's diet can do wonders in eliminating and preventing digestive problems. Garlic helps the intestines function properly, and can also be used to treat inflammation of the gastric canal should digestive complications arise. Consider adding garlic to your favorite dishes, or consuming a teaspoon daily to maintain a healthy digestive system.

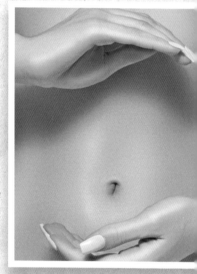

Improve digestive health

PREVENT ALZHEIMER'S AND DEMENTIA

Dementia and Alzheimer's are both terrible neurodegenerative diseases, meaning they degrade the brain over time until it can no longer function properly. Garlic can be used to prevent these diseases due to its antioxidant and anti-inflammatory properties.

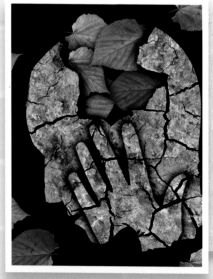

Prevent Alzheimer's

Incorporating it into your diet may stop the inflammation and forming of plaque, preventing the degradation of the brain as one ages.

CONTROL ASTHMA

While it should not be used as a replacement for prescribed asthma medication, garlic can be a used as a supplementary way to control the symptoms of asthma, making asthma attacks less common and making everyday breathing a little easier. Try boiling several cloves of garlic and straining the juice

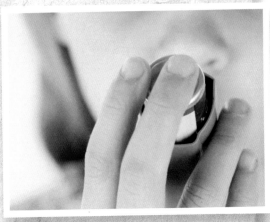

Reduce asthma symptoms

into a glass of milk at night. Drinking this before you go to sleep should reduce the inflammation that can cause your throat to swell up, allowing you to breathe and sleep peacefully.

TREATS URINARY TRACT AND KIDNEY INFECTIONS

One of the primary causes of chronic urinary tract and kidney infections is a bacterium known as *Pseudomonas aeruginosa,* which can cause inflammation and sepsis when it infects your body. Garlic has powerful antibacterial properties, which can help kill harmful bacteria in your body before an infection can set in. Because garlic also reduces inflammation, it will help reduce the pain and discomfort of an infection while the healing process takes place.

WARNING! Be sure not to spray garlic near anything your pets might eat or ingest, as garlic can be toxic to cats, dogs, and other small animals.

USE AS A PESTICIDE IN YOUR GARDEN

Garlic is great at killing bacteria, but it's also useful for keeping insects and other pests away from your flowerbeds. All you need to do is infuse a few bulbs of crushed garlic in a jar or pot of boiling water, leaving it to sit covered for several hours, and then transfer the solution into a spray bottle. Spray this pesticide anywhere you want to keep insects and pests away.

USE AS A GLUE

Because garlic juice forms a natural adhesive when it is released, you can use it as an organic, non-toxic glue for crafts, minor repairs, and other finicky jobs that require a little bit of glue. It generally won't be waterproof, so make sure not to use it on anything that you expect to get wet or damp if you want it to stick for a long time.

GARLIC WELLNESS

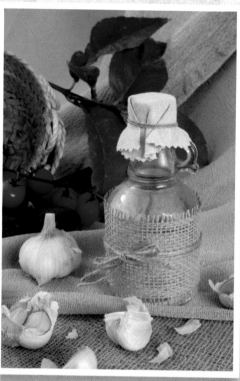

Clean surfaces

MAKE A DIY SURFACE CLEANER

To add some antibacterial power to your DIY cleaning solution, add a few cloves of chopped or ground garlic to a spray bottle full of equal parts white vinegar and lemon juice. This should produce a powerful, natural all-purpose cleaner that will be gentle enough for most surfaces while still killing harmful bacteria and dissolving accumulated dirt and grime.

MINIMIZE ENLARGED PORES

The pores on your face are vital to your skin's health, as they allow you to expel toxins from your body through sweat. They can, however, also lead to breakouts and blackheads when they become clogged by dirt, oil, or dead skin. As you grow older, your pores tend to grow larger, which makes them more noticeable and more easily blocked by debris, which puts you at a greater risk of breakouts and infections. You can use garlic to keep your pores small by making a facial mask of fresh garlic and tomatoes. Mash 4 cloves garlic and ½ a tomato into a smooth paste and apply it liberally to your skin before rinsing it off 20–30 minutes later. Over time, this will soften and exfoliate your skin, shrinking your pores and keeping your face clean and free of blackheads.

HELPS IN REMOVING STRETCH MARKS

Stretch marks are a natural occurrence, appearing whenever your body grows or changes quickly, such as after a growth spurt or during pregnancy. If you want to minimize

Fight stretch marks

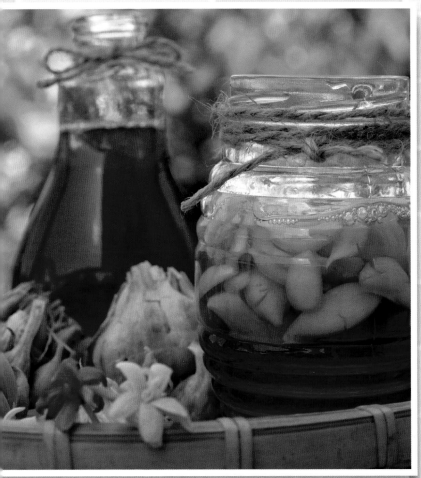

Garlic oil

the appearance of stretch marks, you can apply warm garlic juice or diluted garlic oil topically to any affected areas to help increase the elasticity of your skin, which will soften the appearance of your stretch marks and help prevent more from appearing in the future.

SHINE NAILS

If your nails are dull, brittle, or if you struggle with managing the symptoms of nail fungus, you can use garlic to return them to their former shine and rid them of any harmful bacteria. Garlic will also help fix any discoloration or yellowing of your fingernails. This one is pretty simple: just rub pulped or mashed garlic on your fingernails for a few minutes or leave it on your fingertips to soak for a little while before washing your hands clean with a gentle soap, and you should start to see results within a day or two. Repeat this daily for the best results.

Shine nails

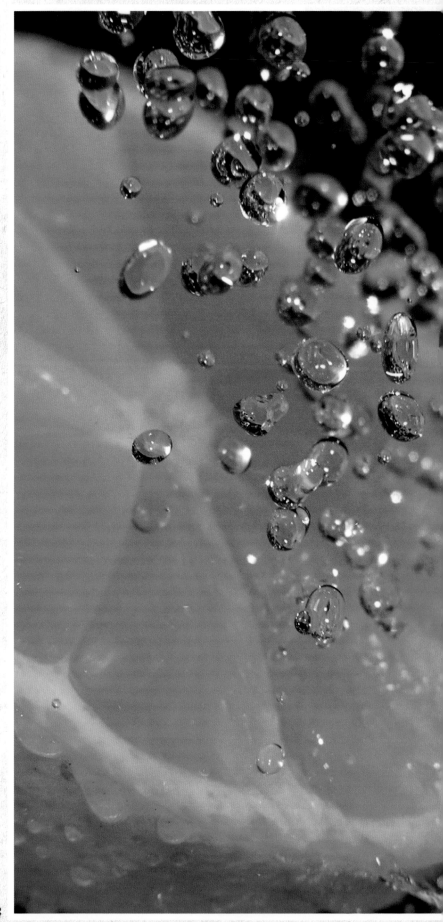

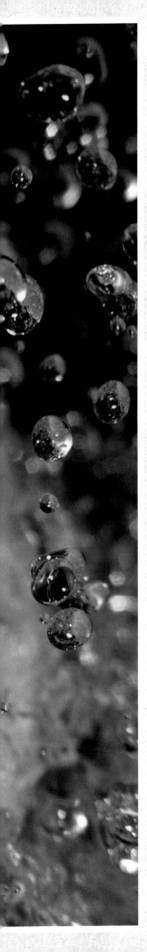

INDEX

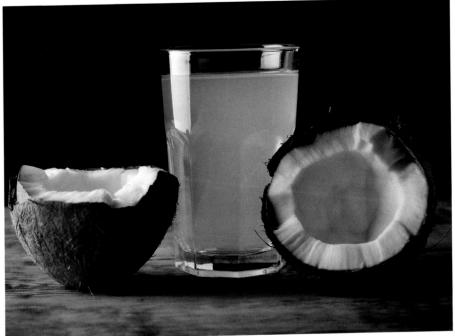

INDEX

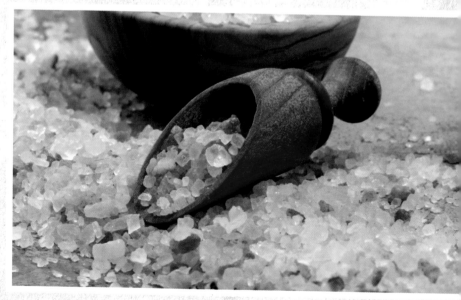

INDEX

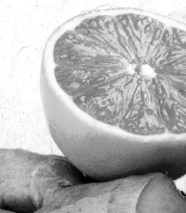

PICTURE CREDITS